THE
HEALTH
EDUCATION
CURRICULUM

THE HEALTH EDUCATION CURRICULUM

A Guide for Curriculum Development in Health Education

J. Keogh Rash, H.S.D., M.P.H.
Indiana University

R. Morgan Pigg, Jr., H.S.D.
University of Georgia

John Wiley & Sons
New York   Chichester   Brisbane   Toronto

Library of Congress Cataloging in Publication Data:

Rash, J   Keogh.
  The health education curriculum.

  Includes bibliographical references and index.
  1.   Health education.   2.   Health education—
Curricula.   I.   Pigg, R. Morgan, joint author.   II.   Title.

RA440.R37   375'.613   78-24493
ISBN 0-471-03765-6

Printed in the United States of America

10 9 8 7 6 5 4 3 2 1

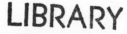

Preface

The critical need for systematic planning in health education, or health science education, has been substantiated and is further emphasized by research studies as well as by word-of-mouth reports on the quality of our health education programs, especially of health instruction. With a few outstanding exceptions, health instruction has been done through textbook teaching with an emphasis on memorizing facts. This extreme dependency on the textbook was reflected in a recent meeting when, after an impassioned plea by the speaker that we plan health instruction according to *pupil needs and interests as revealed by class discussions and surveys*, the first question to the speaker was "what is the best textbook?"

In connection with the study of aims and objectives, it was a common practice of one of my former professors to hand someone in class a five dollar bill and say "Go buy me a railway ticket." Of course the common reply was, "Where do you want to go?" That is still the question in health education, and it can only be answered at the local level in terms of the needs and interests of the students concerned. This demands local planning; curriculum, courses of study, units, and lessons, and this planning must involve all those concerned with the health and welfare of students, including the students themselves.

The purpose of this book is to provide guidelines for the health educator who is concerned with developing the health education curriculum. Curriculum development in any subject matter area is a complicated process. In health education it is further complicated by the diverse nature of the curriculum, by the controversial nature of some of the problem areas, and by the many disciplines and agencies that contribute to the process of health education and, hence, to the curriculum. It is not the purpose of this textbook to deal extensively with theories of curriculum development. However, the general principles of curriculum development, as applied to health education, may be applicable in other curricular areas.

The concept of health education, as presented in this book, is a broad range concept embodying all aspects of the school health program. In fact, it would be more accurate to refer to the school health education program rather than the school health program.

It is the thesis of this presentation that all aspects of the school health program should be, primarily, educational in nature and that, with few exceptions, unless a service rendered by the school is basically educational it probably has no place in the school program.

This textbook is a revised, updated, and enlarged version of a book that has been used by the senior author in his health education curriculum classes and in similar classes elsewhere. The authors acknowledge with sincere appreciation the contributions that have been made by the hundreds of students who have used the book. Their questions, criticisms, and suggestions have helped in the attempt to develop a textbook that may be helpful in the long haul of constantly improving the health education curriculum.

The three parts of the book are intended to serve different purposes as indicated by the titles. Part 1 provides a historical, philosophical, theoretical, and pragmatic foundation for developing the curriculum in health and safety education. Part 2 provides some guidelines in the realm of curriculum engineering, how to go about organizing the school and community for the project and procedures in developing the curriculum. Part 3 provides some specific suggestions regarding the health education curriculum at each of the major developmental levels, including college and adult populations. A few examples of partial instructional units are included. These are not intended to be ideal or complete units. They are intended to be used as guidelines for developing units based on the local circumstances and the criteria for selecting expected outcomes and content for the local community. They are not intended to serve as actual teaching units for any locality. To suggest such use would be to violate the basic principles of curriculum development that this textbook espouses.

While every effort has been made to give full credit for material drawn from other sources, the principal source for the basis for this textbook has been the course in *Health Education Curriculum* as originally developed and taught for several years by Willard W. Patty in the School of Health, Physical Education, and Recreation, Indiana University. Credit is hereby given for any material drawn unwittingly and without acknowledgement from other sources.

J. Keogh Rash
R. Morgan Pigg, Jr.

vi

Contents

CONTENTS

Firm in the belief that one's philosophy is the foundation of behavior, we submit the following statement of beliefs regarding health and health education. It is hoped that these statements will be of assistance to health educators, and prospective health educators, in developing their own philosophy to guide and sustain them in their pursuit of a life of service and satisfaction in their chosen profession.

My School Health Creed

I believe the total health of the pupil is the most important concern of the school.

I believe the school health program is the most important program of the school.

I believe the health education of the pupil is the most important obligation of the school.

I believe the goal of health education is intelligent self-direction of health behavior.

I believe every aspect of the school program can contribute to the health education of the pupil.

I believe a concentrated health education course facilitates the functional integration of diverse health education experience.

I believe planned coordination is essential to an effective school health program.

Compiled by Members of the Department of Health and Safety Education; School of Health, Physical Education, and Recreation
Indiana University

THE
HEALTH
EDUCATION
CURRICULUM

PART ONE
HEALTH
EDUCATION
CURRICULUM
FOUNDATIONS

Chapter One

Historical Foundations of Health Education

The human concern for the conservation of health probably antedates recorded history. As is true of the lower forms of animal life, much of human behavior that may be classed as health conservation is *instinctive*, and much is *acquired* through the learning process as a result of experience. In many instances the learning is the result of direct personal experiences, often disagreeable or painful. However, as effective methods of preserving knowledge and effective means of communication developed, it has become possible to acquire vast amounts of knowledge and, hopefully, to influence behavior through the indirect experiences of others. Only in rare instances is the actual, first-hand, experience now a necessary basis for learning. In the phenomenon of learning the developing individual follows a pattern quite similar to that followed by the human race in its learning. One of the principles of biology is expressed in the saying, *ontogeny recapitulates phylogeny*. In many respects the same can be said about learning. To a very great extent the learning pattern of a human being, from birth to maturity, recapitulates the learning experiences of the human race.

In fetal life, in infancy, and then in early childhood, learning is achieved almost exclusively through direct experiences. Soon direct learning may be associated with verbal or visual symbols of approval or disapproval, in such a way that these and other symbols may be substituted for the actual experience itself. With growth and development toward maturation the necessity for direct experience is generally reduced. As we mature we become able to better deal with abstract ideas and we are better able to see associations or relationships that make it possible for us to understand and often predict cause-and-effect relationships. To the extent that this predictability becomes possible we can rely less on personal, direct experiences as the basis for learning and more on abstract reasoning and the reports of the experiences of others, even those of recorded history.

3

We have reached a time in the development of *homo sapiens* and of mature human beings when much of the health conservation behavior can be learned as a result of the application of knowledge that has been acquired through previous experience, preserved, and passed on to subsequent generations. While it is, indeed, most fortunate that we have reached this stage of development, this too presents some problems of communication and learning that have not been solved. As Turner indicated,

> *The need for planned and effective health education in this rapidly changing world, with new health problems, new possibilities of health promotion, cultural change, urban migration, industrialization, and new way of living, is crystal clear. (14:3)*

One of the most important problems in this connection is to determine what are the most important knowledges and practices related to the conservation of health. A second and equally important problem is how to make certain that all human beings are aware of those important knowledges and practices. These two problems probably constitute the foundation of the health education program as we know it today. Thus the test of the effectivenes of the program is the extent to which all persons come in contact with and use those health knowledges and practices that are important for them.

Early Efforts in Health Education

The earliest recorded efforts to influence health behavior through education took place in early Biblical times. Such success as was attained, for example, in the prevention of communicable diseases such as trichinosis and leprosy, was the result of codes of behavior that grew out of human experience as observed by the leaders. These observations were handed from generation to generation by the chief educational institution of the time, the church. Subsequent history records efforts, both successful and unsuccessful, to achieve an effective level of health conservation. As is true of most progress, progress in health conservation has been achieved through successes and failures, gains and losses, moving ahead and slipping back—in many instances gaining a little more than was lost, until the long perspective of history reveals that we have, in fact, made remarkable progress.

From time to time a special effort has been made to promote the conservation of health. The Hellas (700–600 B.C.) were devoted to developing a high level of physical fitness and to the conservation of health through practices then thought to be desirable. Such individuals as Comenius (1592–1670), John Locke (1632–1704), Rousseau (1712–1778), Basedow (1723–1790), Guts Muths (1759–1839), and Horace Mann (1796–1859) provided early leadership that served to focus on health and the importance of health education. The following early move-

4

ments or events, all of which took place before 1900, are milestones in the development of the health education program.

Bavaria free lunch to the underprivileged (1790)

U.S. Merchant Seaman's Act (1798), which later became the U.S. Public Health Service

Sanitary school laws in France (1833 and 1842)

German Gymnastic Society (1848)

Shattuck Report, Massachusetts (1850), that laid the foundation for our public health program

Founding of the American Public Health Association (1870)

Doctors placed on the school staff of public schools in Sweden (1868), Germany (1869), Russia (1871), Austria (1873), and Belgium (1874)

Regular medical inspection in schools in Brussels (1874)

School kitchens established in Boston by Mrs. Ellen Richards (1887)

School nursing in London started by Amy Hughes (1891)

Medical inspection in Boston schools initiated by Dr. Samuel Durgin (1894) and introduced into the schools of Chicago (1895), New York (1897) and Philadelphia (1898)

The Wiesbaden Plan (1896) of physical examinations of students

Connecticut law requiring the testing of eyesight (1899)

School nurse added to the school staff in New York City, under the leadership of Lillian Walk (1899)

Health instruction, as such, made its first appearance in American schools as requirements for the teaching of the harmful effects of alcohol, drugs, and narcotics. Considerable impetus was given to this kind of teaching by such organizations as the Women's Christian Temperance Union, founded in 1874. Under the leadership of Frances Willard, President from 1879–1898, the WCTU developed its temperance education program, which played an important role in the school health (hygiene) education program for at least 35 years.

A White House Conference on Children and Youth has been held every 10 years since 1909, when President Theodore Roosevelt convened the first such conference. Each conference considered a different problem, the first being concerned with the Care of Dependent Children. According to Means, the 1930 White House Conference on Child Health and Protection was especially important to the development of school health education. (4:90–91)

The school health instruction program as we know it first began near the end of World War I, in 1918. Since that time the educational emphasis has shifted from classes that were physiologically oriented to those that emphasized healthful living as a means of conserving health.

The transition from a concern only for the physical health of the school child to that of its total welfare, including health education, came very slowly. Three prominent leaders in education gave impetus to this idea. Henry Barnard (1811–1900) was interested in the health aspects of school buildings (4:72), and Horace Mann (1796–1859) was an early proponent of physical education, including emphasis on health education. (4:32–33) William Holmes McGuffey (1800–1873), through his famous *Eclectic Readers*, emphasized good health practices, including the area of mental health.

Means reported that Harvard and Amherst Colleges vie for the distinction of providing the first health instruction classes in the early 1800s. (4:375) Mount Holyoke, Smith, Wellesley, and Vassar were also among the colleges to provide health (hygiene) instruction by 1850. Those programs usually included physical activities (called physical training) as well as physiology and anatomy. (4:375)

The cooperative efforts of the American Medical Association and the National Education Association deserve recognition. Established in 1911 under the leadership of Thomas D. Wood, M.D., the Joint Committee on Health Problems in Education of the National Education Association and the American Medical Association has encouraged the joint efforts of the two associations in implementing total school health programs. The two associations have worked together through subcommittees; joint efforts in meetings; through such publications as *Health Education*, (6) first published in 1924; *School Health Services*, (16) first published in 1953; *Healthful School Living* (17) (*Healthful School Environment*), first published in 1957; numerous other publications; and the Bi-ennial Conference on Physicians and Schools. The publication *Suggested School Health Policies* (7) has also been a helpful guide for school health programs since its first publication in 1940. Even though the Joint Committee has been disbanded, the American Medical Association has continued its interest in health education through the creation of an interdisciplinary medical education committee.

Immediately following World War I several health education projects were undertaken. Four five-year demonstration projects were organized and financed by the Commonwealth Fund (4:168–169). These were in Fargo, North Dakota (1923–1927); Rutherford County, Tennessee (1924–1928); Clarke County, Athens, Georgia (1924–1928); and Marion County, Salem, Oregon (1925–1929). The demonstrations included special emphasis on an educational program in the school as well as coordination of the health agencies in the communities. These projects demonstrated that health education could be an effective school- community undertaking.

Means (4:296–298) described the School-Community Health Project sponsored by the W. K. Kellogg Foundation. This project originated in Michigan in 1942 and was expanded to include some 24 states, which received grants for it

6

over a three-year period. California, Illinois, Nebraska, Ohio, and Texas were selected for continued assistance for three more years. The purpose of the programs was to study and improve the effectiveness of school (college and university)-community cooperation as well as coordination within an institution. The services of a coordinator were made available to work in the institution and in coordinating the programs of the institutions and the community.

The School Health Education Study directed by Elena M. Sliepcevich (11) and financed by the Bronfman Foundation was the most ambitious study so far undertaken; it has had a profound effect on school health instruction programs. Beginning in 1961, the study surveyed instructional practices in a large sampling of schools and subsequently conducted health behavior inventories in some 1101 elementary schools and 359 secondary schools in 38 states. Upon completion of the study the project was continued as a Curriculum Development Project under the sponsorship of the Minnesota Mining and Manufacturing Company (3M). The culmination of this project was the publication of a proposed health education curriculum based on the conceptual approach and subsequent teaching materials published by the 3M Education Press (Chapter 13).

In the professional preparation of health educators, Teachers College of Columbia University and Harvard–Massachusetts Institute of Technology rank among the pioneers. Under the leadership of Thomas D. Wood, M.D., Columbia University provided some of the earliest professional preparation in health education, granting the first undergraduate degree in health education in 1922. (5:197). The Harvard–M.I.T. program, under the direction of Clair E. Turner, Dr. P.H. (1890–1976), in the school year of 1921–1922 offered the first course in health education ever offered in a School of Public Health. (13:72)

Health education soon began to be a regular offering in other Schools of Public Health, notably Harvard, Yale, Michigan, University of California at Berkeley, and Minnesota. In about the same period, 1925–1940, other universities began offering courses, and finally degrees, in school health education. In addition to Columbia University, professional preparation in health education was offered early in New York University, Stanford University, Indiana University, University of Colorado, University of Alabama, West Virginia University, and others.

Indiana University was a pioneer in establishing a separate autonomous School of Health, Physical Education, and Recreation. In 1939, by vote of the University Faculty, Indiana University approved a School of Health, Physical Education, and Recreation. Under the leadership of W. W. Patty, Ph.D., the School was organized and accepted the first students in the fall of 1946. The unique feature of the School was the three separate and autonomous departments of Health and Safety Education, Physical Education, and Recreation and Park Administration. About the same time West Virginia University also established a similar School.

7

The pattern of organization of a School—with a Department of Health Education, Health and Safety Education, or Health Science—has been widely accepted since about 1950. This has given health education a distinct identity, entirely separate from and independent of its parent, physical education. The separation into the two distinct disciplines has strengthened both and has given each of them a well-deserved identity.

In the earlier days of offering health education, credit was not always granted for the course. As Means (4:286) pointed out, by 1940 health education was beginning to be a recognized subject in the curriculum.

With the emphasis on health education in the public elementary schools following World War I, it became common practice to offer a health course in each grade with a textbook of appropriate content and reading difficulty. Since it was the general practice to attempt to cover most all of the health problem areas in each textbook, the students soon began to feel that they were studying the same things over and over again each year. This feeling of repetition and the criticism that accompanied it soon gave impetus to the cycle plan, which will be discussed in Chapter 10.

As we have been able to discover, the *cycle plan* of instruction made its first appearance in the 1933 State Course of Study for Elementary Schools in the State of Indiana (12) (Figure 1). Dr. W. W. Patty, former Dean of the School of Health, Physical Education, and Recreation, Indiana University, was active in the development of the 1933 State Course of Study for Indiana. Dr. Patty also proposed a cycle plan for health instruction in elementary grades in his book *Teaching Health and Safety in Elementary Grades* (9:4–5), which was first published in 1940.

The first statewide application of the cycle plan in grades one to twelve came with the development of Oregon's Four-Cycle Health Curriculum that was introduced into the Oregon schools during the 1945–46 school year. This curriculum was described by Dr. Hoyman (2:223–224) in an article that appeared in *The Journal of Health and Physical Education* in April, 1947. This plan has undergone considerable modification since it was first adopted, but it still retains the cycle principle.

Safety education has long been recognized as a vital responsibility of both the home and the school. It is probably the first general concern of parents toward the welfare of the infant. Similarly it is one of the first concerns of school personnel, with special attention focused on the playground. Because of the direct impact on health of injuries resulting from accidents, health education efforts have generally included an emphasis on safety. The relationship between safety education and health education is so close that the term health education commonly includes general safety education. However, it does not ordinarily include such specialized safety instruction as driver education or industrial safety

8

Grades (The order of units in each grade is not fixed)		
I Nutrition	Safety and first aid	Personal Cleanliness
II Fresh air, sunshine, exercise, and respiration	Mental and emotional health	Control of communicable diseases
III Clothing, including shoes	Care of nose, ears, eyes, throat, and voice	Safety and first aid
IV Nutrition	Temperance	Personal Cleanliness
V Fresh air, sunshine exercise, and respiration	Temperance	Clothing, including shoes
VI Control of communicable diseases	Temperance	Nutrition
VII Mental and emotional health	Temperance	Safety and first aid
VIII Care of nose, ears, eyes, throat, and voice	Temperance	Control of communicable diseases

Figure 1. Indiana Cycle Plan (1933) State of Indiana, Department of Public Instruction, Bulletin No. 107F, *Tentative Course of Study in Physical and Health Education,* 1933.

education. In instances where the reference extends beyond general safety education the expression "health and safety education" is used.

The shift of emphasis from physiology to healthful living has served to make health instruction more applicable to meeting health needs but, at the same time, it may have given health instruction a less than favorable academic respectability. In fact, the shift from memorization of parts and functions of the body to the application of such knowledge should, in reality, increase the significance of the learning. In a changing environment a deeper and more significant understanding is fundamental to the proper application of the knowledge than is possible from pure memorization. However, we should avoid reducing teaching to the ineffective memorization of slogans, rules, and knowledge of desirable practices and, instead, inculcate the attitudes and habits that will insure desirable behavior.

Does the progress that has been made in health mean that we have outgrown the need for health education? Has civilization progressed to the point where the accumulation of health conservation practices is adequate for meeting the health needs of the population in this time? Although the obvious answer is no, why? A quick review of the health conditions pertaining to mental illness, alcoholism, heart and circulatory disorders, cancer, venereal diseases, dental caries, ac-

9

cidents, tuberculosis and other respiratory diseases, the inadequate immunization level of the population, and pollution of lakes, rivers, and air, to mention some of the more acute problems, quickly reminds us that the job is not done. The answer is all the more confusing and frustrating when we realize that we actually possess enough knowledge of each of the conditions mentioned to solve that health problem. Therefore, since we know the answers, why do the problems persist? They persist, in part, as the result of human weakness, the influences of peer pressure, the lack of self-discipline, and the refusal to accept the responsibility for ordering one's life to be able to benefit from the vast body of available knowledge.

In health conservation, society has done for the individual just about all that it can do; it remains for individuals to *do for themselves*. They must utilize the health knowledge that is now readily available. Therefore the *process of health education* (health instruction) must take a place. Individuals must be taught to direct their own health behavior in a manner that will best conserve their health and thus improve the quality of their lives. Such self-direction comes about only as a result of successful health education.

But what is health education, and what is the role of the health educator in the health conservation picture? A partial answer to the question can be found in considering the professional school health educator. What does the school health educator do? What preparation or skills are needed? What are some of the special frustrations and some of the rewards of the job?

What Is Health Education?

Thomas D. Wood defined health education as

the sum of experiences in school and elsewhere that favorably influence habits, attitudes, and knowledge relating to individual, community, and racial health (18:1)

Such a definition suggests the many ramifications of the educational process are intended to achieve these results. This process, with all its ramifications, creates the need for considering the health education curriculum.

For many years the Committee on Terminology (1:14) defined the process of health education as

the process of providing learning experiences for the purpose of influencing knowledges, attitudes, and conduct relating to individual and group health. (1:14)

While these two definitions of health are in general agreement, Dr. Wood's definition is more general and reflects the concept of several different kinds of ex-

10

periences in school and elsewhere that may favorably influence behavior, whereas the definition of the Committee on Terminology refers a little more specifically to the process of *providing learning experiences* in school. This emphasis might be considered *instruction*, whether it takes place in the classroom, or school, or elsewhere.

The Joint Committee on Health Education Terminology released a definition of health education that merits consideration. According to that definition, health education is

a process with intellectual, psychological, and social dimensions relating to activities which increase the abilities of people to make informed decisions affecting their personal, family, and community well being. This process, based on scientific principles, facilitates learning and behavioral change in both health personnel and consumers, including children and youth (3:25–30)

For our purposes the term *health education* includes all experiences that may influence the individual in matters of health. When referring to the teaching program, usually in school but not limited to the school, we will use the term health instruction.

Although the development of the curriculum is logically the responsibility of the school and school personnel, the involvement of nonschool personnel may be beneficial to the school program, as will be emphasized later.

Who Is the Health Educator?

Having identified health education, let us now consider who is responsible for it. Wood has suggested that it takes place "in the school and elsewhere." (18:1) He thus foresaw the two branches of health education in existence today, school health education and public (community) health education; the principal differentiating factor is where the process takes place. Since the place will, quite naturally, automatically create or prescribe certain conditions, there will be differences in procedures. Nevertheless, there will be many things in common. The characteristics of the health education programs in these two settings are discussed more fully in the section "The School in the Community Health Program," Chapter 6.

It is an old, and much overworked, adage that every teacher is a health teacher; nevertheless, it does contain some truth. It is also true that every teacher is an English teacher, or that every teacher is a mathematics teacher, or a science teacher. If the job of educators is the fullest possible development of the total individual, then every teacher must make use of the opportunities to contribute to

11

the total development of the individual in any and every way the teacher's particular abilities permit. This dictates that health instruction be provided when the opportunity is present, not just when the class is scheduled. This does not preclude or minimize the class, of course, because the class provides a special opportunity for instruction. It does mandate that other opportunities be used as they appear, or are made to appear.

Although many people share in the health education process, not everyone who does some health teaching can be classified as a health educator. The health educator is a special person, with a specialized background of education uniquely equipping him or her for the task of providing health instruction and of fostering the process of health education in the several aspects of the school program.

The background of educational preparation of the health educator should include a major in health education, or health and safety education, with additional preparation in the life sciences, the behavioral and social sciences, and in educational methodology. The minimum preparation should be a minor of at least 24 semester hours in health and safety education, with a good background in the other areas mentioned.

The personal qualifications of the health educator should include a strong interest in health conservation through education, a genuine interest in and concern for others, a desire to keep up-to-date on professional matters, and the willingness and ability to change as knowledge advances but not just for the sake of change. The health educator, perhaps more than any other teacher, must be able to communicate effectively—in a manner that will motivate to action.

What is the Role of the Health Educator?

In the typical school or college situation the health educator will teach one or more health classes. He or she will probably carry other responsibilities for promoting a coordinated school health program. These may include serving as a health coordinator; serving on the school health committee; directing and/or supervising health education curriculum development projects; providing individual, personal, health counsel and guidance to students, staff, faculty, and administration; and, on occasion discussing health problems with parents or other appropriate community representatives.

Three special responsibilities are inherent in teaching; in fact they may constitute the chief responsibilities of the teacher. These are *motivating, clarifying,* and *informing.* Motivation is undoubtedly the prime responsibility of the health educator. In addition, the health educator must be able to interpret and clarify questions and problems and be able to introduce new knowledge when it becomes available.

Dr. Marjorie Young, (19) of the Harvard School of Public Health, has labeled these functions the Three I's of Methodology:

Inspiration—Motivating

Interpretation—Clarifying and explaining

Information—Informing

In addition to the three I's, the teacher has the responsibility for promoting a favorable physical, social, and emotional climate. This includes concern for heating, lighting, ventilation, seating, personal relationships of all concerned, and a regimen that helps reduce fatigue to a minimum and that provides opportunities for self-realization along with concern for others.

This perception of the role of the teacher suggests a new definition of teaching. Teaching is defined as *fostering an environment that is conducive to learning.* For too long a time teaching has been erroneously considered and described as imparting knowledge. In fact, little if any knowledge can be passed to another person. The learner is the key individual. It is the learner who accepts, adopts, and uses any knowledge made available. The environment will be more conducive to learning if there is *proper motivation, adequate explanation* of points not otherwise made clear, and *introduction of new or additional information* that might not otherwise be available to the learner.

The learning process takes place within the individual. One can be exposed to knowledge, attitudes, and practices, but rarely can one be directly made to learn, and less to practice what one has been exposed to. Because health education is concerned predominantly with sound attitudes and practices, the health educator has a particularly difficult task: to cultivate attitudes and practices that are often vigorously resisted by the learner. This is precisely the reason why a subtle approach is needed. In teaching that involves knowledge a direct, frontal approach may be used, whereas in health instruction attempts to modify behavior may immediately bring resistance. The extent to which this is true varies with individuals depending, in part, on the fixation of the attitude or practice involved.

It is reasonable to assume that desirable health attitudes and practices are as easy to inculcate as undesirable ones if they were taught from the beginning. The chief difficulty appears when it becomes necessary to break or unlearn an old habit (e.g., of attitude or of practice) and then to instill a new one. The difference in success in establishing a habit depends little, if any, on whether the habit is desirable or undesirable. The success in establishing a desirable versus an undesirable practice depends on which is the easier or more natural to learn and on which gives the greater satisfaction at a time when the person is most receptive to learning.

13

The special responsibility of the health educator is to influence health behavior by stengthening positive practices and fostering the substitution of positive for negative practices. The task has to do with applied psychology. However, any such responsibility must have its foundation in scientifically sound facts about health. Hence, the health educator needs a background in the life and the behavioral sciences, in addition to a sound basic preparation in health and health education. The health educator should understand health-threatening behavior, the motivations for enhancing health behavior (e.g., personal threat), and theories regarding preventive health action. Knowledge of the theories regarding attitude and behavior change is mandatory, hence, the emphasis on the behavioral sciences. Furthermore, from the rich background of educational experiences certain procedures of instruction have been found to be effective, and the health educator needs to have all possible effective teaching (instructional) techniques available.

In actual practice the health educator is faced with the dilemma of frustrations and satisfactions. Frustrations result from the realization that results are not always apparent. Knowing does not guarantee doing, and neither does the resolution to practice desirable health practices guarantee consistent compliance. Often the health educator will not get, or see, the desired results. However, the satisfaction of seeing some favorable results offsets the frustrations of apparent failure. The learner who *does* what is desirable for the conservation of health is a real joy to the person who has been instrumental in bringing about the results. In such cases the benefits are twofold: immediate satisfaction to the health educator *and* continuing satisfaction (and health conservation) to the learner.

References

1. Committee on Terminology in School Health Education, *The Journal of the American Association for Health, Physical Education and Recreation*, 22: 7 (1951).

2. Hoyman, H.S., "Oregon's Four Cycle Health Curriculum," *Journal of Health and Physical Education*, 18: 4 (1947).

3. Joint Committee on Health Education Terminology, *School Health Review*, 4: 6 (1973).

4. Means, R.K., *A History of Health Education in the United States*, Lea & Febiger, Philadelphia, 1962.

5. Means, R.K., *Historical Perspectives on School Health*, Slack, Thorofare, New Jersey, 1975.

6. Moss, B.R., Editor, *Health Education*, National Education Association, Washington, D.C., 1961.

7. National Committee on School Health Policies of the National Education Association and the American Medical Association, *Suggested School Health Policies*, Fourth Edition, American Medical Association, Chicago, 1966.

8. Nyswander, D.B., *Solving School Health Problems*, Commonwealth Fund, Oxford University Press, London, 1942.

9. Patty, W.W., *Teaching Health and Safety in Elementary Grades*, Prentice-Hall, New York, 1940.

10. Russell, R.D., *Health Education*, National Education Association, Washington, D.C., 1975.

11. Sliepcevich, E.M., *School Health Education Study, A Summary Report*, School Health Education Study, Washington, D.C., 1964.

12. State of Indiana, *Tentative Course of Study in Physical and Health Education, Grades One to Eight*, Department of Public Instruction, Indianapolis, 1933.

13. Turner, C.E., *I Remember*, Vantage, New York, 1974.

14. Turner, C.E., *Planning for Health Education, UNESCO Source Book*, Longmans, London, 1966.

15. U.S. Department of HEW, *Child Health in America*, Rockville, Maryland, 1976.

16. Wilson, C.C., Editor, *School Health Services*, National Education Association and the American Medical Association, Washington, D.C., 1964.

17. Wilson, C.C. and E.A. Wilson, Editors, *Healthful School Living*, National Education Association and the American Medical Association, Washington, D.C., 1969.

18. Wood, T.D. and M.O. Lerrigo, *Health Behavior*, Public School Publishing Co., Bloomington, Illinois, 1928.

19. Young, M.A.C., "The Learning Process," a talk delivered to the Kentucky School Health Workshop, Cumberland Falls, Kentucky, June 7, 1960.

Chapter Two
Philosophical Bases for Health Education

The philosophy of the individual is the foundation of all human behavior. In light of modern psychology, especially of behavioristic psychology, such a bold statement raises several questions. First, what do we mean by philosophy? It would be difficult and too time-consuming to explore all possible meanings of the word philosophy, but the number of concepts of philosophy may be reduced to a workable minimum if we approach the matter from the point of view of *my philosophy*. This approach rules out the use of the term philosophy if it refers to an academic discipline as well as a historical approach to the study of philosophy. However, other differing concepts remain.

Recognizing that other, usually more complex, definitions of philosophy do exist, and for some purposes are more acceptable, we proposed, as a basis for this discussion, that *one's philosophy is what one believes.* In this respect there may be a significant divergence between what one *knows* and what one *believes.*

There is abundant support in curriculum literature for the belief that the values held by the members of a community, their philosophy, serves as the foundation of the curriculum. Early writers such as Smith, Stanley, and Shores (15), and Bobbitt (4) proposed this idea. It is also strongly supported by current writers such as Beauchamp (5), Goodlad (11), and Tyler (17).

If it is true that one's philosophy is the foundation of individual behavior, then it becomes vitally important that health education efforts be grounded in a sound philosophy of health and health education. You, as a health educator, may be motivated and, hopefully, assisted in developing your own satisfactory and ef-

* This chapter is based on an article by Rash that was published in *The Journal of Health, Physical Education, and Recreation, 31,* 1, (1960). Used with permission of The American Alliance for Health, Physical Education, and Recreation.

fective philosophy of health and health education, by the following definitions of health.

In one of the early and most widely quoted definitions, Williams defined health as that condition of the organism which enables one to "live most and serve best." (16:12) Some years later the Joint Committee on Health Problems in Education of the National Education Association and the American Medical Association (13:38) emphasized the physical, mental, and spiritual possibilities of the individual. The World Health Organization (WHO) defined health as complete physical, mental, and social well-being, and not merely freedom from disease or infirmity. (6:29–34)

In contrast to these definitions of health, disease has been defined as

a physiological or psychological disequilibrium state leading to cellular or organism discomfort, disability, or death. (1:15)

Such a definition may be adequate as a definition of disease, but it tells us very little about health.

Although each of these definitions of health has merit each has shortcomings. Williams' definition proposes a very noble goal, but it tells us very little about the nature of health. The WHO definition has three shortcomings. (1) It sets the unattainable goal of *complete well-being.* (2) The term *mental* generally refers to the intellect or intelligence. (3) It omits any reference to the intangible or non-material aspects of life.

Our fourfold definition of health allows for perfection (completeness) of well-being when possible, but does not exclude the person for whom that perfection is not possible. It embodies the concept of levels of wellness, as proposed by Dunn. (9) Instead of complete well-being we are proposing *optimum* well-being. This means the well-being that is best for the individual. Also we use the term *emotional* instead of mental and we are including *spiritual*, as suggested by the Joint Committee. (13) *Health is optimum physical, emotional, social, and spiritual well-being.* This is the concept that will be used throughout the textbook. Hoyman gave support to the concept of spiritual well-being when he said "the four pathways to health are a sound body, an alert mind, a compassionate heart, and a creative spirit." (12:279) Bauer (3:35) gave equivalent support to this concept when he pointed out the importance of a satisfactory spiritual life in times of stress and turmoil.

The Fourfold Nature of Health

If we analyze the definitions of health in terms of the four aspects we find that *physical well-being* may be considered the condition of the organism that permits activity without undue fatigue and in which the organism is free from disease or

18

disability. *Emotional well-being* is the condition of the organism that enables one to satisfactorily meet the day-to-day emotional experiences of life, such as joy, sorrow, success, disappointment, fear, and courage. It provides the balance wheel, or gyroscope, for the daily emotional stresses. *Spiritual well-being* enables the organism to meet and deal satisfactorily with the nonmaterial aspects of life such as the infinite, the supernatural, life, death, and eternity. As Hoyman pointed out "[s]piritual and ethical values are central to human personality development and mental health; but faith alone will not make a person healthy or more fully human." (12:279) Spiritual well-being is dependent, in part, on an *inner peace* that stems from both faith and the cultivation of a guiding inner light. *Social well-being* is that condition of the organism that enables one to associate with her or his fellows easily, pleasantly, and with personal satisfaction to both the individual and the associates. It is concerned with interpersonal relationships and depends in part on a social consciousness, effective communication, and concern for the welfare of others.

To illustrate this fourfold nature of health, let us visualize health as a wheel or circle. Divide the wheel into four parts, and let each part represent one of the four phases of health: physical, emotional, spiritual, and social. If the various parts are viewed separately, each part represents a sector of a circle. As long as the parts of the wheel remain together and in symmetry, the wheel is balanced and may be rolled smoothly and accurately. Loss of symmetry results in an imbalance that symbolizes a state of disequilibrium, or disease.

Symmetrical Development

In this age of speed, it is not difficult to realize that a ball must be symmetrical if it is to have any degree of equilibrium or stability. The importance of a balanced wheel, or the hazard of imbalance, on a high-speed automobile is realized by most people. Before basketballs were molded, both manufacturers and players were aware of the problem of symmetry and balance. Manufacturers today emphasize the symmetry they have been able to achieve and consistently maintain throughout the manufacturing process. This picture is not unlike the health picture for an individual. Failure to maintain symmetry or equilibrium through neglect of any aspect of health (physical, emotional, spiritual, or social), results in an unbalanced life. The individual may crack under the stress of life, especially if the stress becomes great enough.

Galdston (10:13) has pointed out the importance of stress and deprivation in health and disease. These factors are directly related to the emotional and spiritual aspects of health. As Bauer aptly stated,

What we need at every age in life is a sane and sensible balance of these three (physical, mental, and spiritual), (3:35) to which we add the fourth, *social.*

19

Symmetry in the sphere of health (equilibrium), as achieved by proper attention to the fourfold development, has become vital as the pace of life continues to increase. In horse-and-buggy days a wheel slightly out of balance was scarcely noticed, but today, in an era of jet propulsion, balance is of vital importance. Failure to give attention to the conservation of any aspect of health jeopardizes a person's well-being. In short, the fourfold nature of health and the importance of each aspect in its relation to total health dictate that each individual must give proper attention to being well-rounded.

Interrelationships of the Four Aspects of Health

It is important that we recognize the interrelatedness of the four aspects of health. No single aspect exists independently of the others. *Physical* well-being is probably most directly dependent on emotional, spiritual, and social well-being. For example, ulcers may result from emotional stress. *Emotional* well-being is closely related to social, spiritual, and often physical well-being. Social problems such as divorce, or a physical illness such as diabetes may well precipitate an emotional illness. *Social* well-being is often dependent on factors that are largely emotional or physical, and sometimes spiritual. A physical problem such as severe acne may impair one's social health. *Spiritual* well-being is closely related to emotional well-being. Emotional stress such as the death of a loved one may impair, or sometimes enhance, spiritual well-being.

The optimum level of health is reached when there is the greatest possible *well-being* of all aspects of health. No one is blessed, for long, with perfect health. As Dubos said "complete freedom from disease and from struggle is almost incompatible with the process of living." (8:13) The ultimate challenge to health educators is to help individuals attain and maintain their optimum levels of health.

Jonas Salk suggested that health may be used to combat disease. He proposed that "[w]hat is needed is means of augmenting and strengthening the forces for health of body, mind, and emotions, and of the constructive and creative part of man, each and all of which require nourishment and exercise to be fully expressed." (14:582–584) He proposed that a good place to start this process is in the schools where the child can begin to develop habits of thinking and behaving that will favor maintenance of a state of health (health conservation).

Importance of Health

Viewed in the light of the previous discussion, health seems to be the most important single aspect of life. For what would you trade your health? In terms of monetary or property value, fame, influence, or prestige, it is impossible to place a value on health. An old Egyptian saying illustrates the importance and general feeling about health:

Health is a Crown upon the well man's head, but no one can see it but a sick man. *

Nothing in life is so taken for granted when possessed, and so sorely missed when lost as is health. This fact suggests a philosophical basis for health education.

If health is so commonly the concern of only the sick, it may be that we are failing to emphasize aspects of health that are challenging to well persons. In speaking of her interest in the study of certain diseases, one high school girl was heard to say,

Of course I wasn't interested in the childhood diseases which I had already had, but I was interested in those diseases which might be a problem to me.

In another vein, perhaps we are not taking advantage of our opportunities to promote the health-educated individual because we fail to take advantage of teachable moments at times of illness. For example, few hospitals and almost no physicians have a health educator on their staff to assist the patient or the family in the solution of health problems, or in living within known limitations.

Hospitals are just beginning to realize the possible favorable impact of a planned patient health education program and are employing educators to run such a program. Such health promotion activities can do much both to assist in the restoration of health and to promote a higher level of health for the patients involved as well as for their families and other close associates.

Being Health Educated

When is one health educated? To answer this question let us first state the goal of health education as suggested by the American Association of School Administrators:

The goal of intelligent self direction of health behavior by every person in our society is an ideal toward which to strive. (2:59)

In other words, if I am health educated, I will be able to intelligently direct my own behavior concerning physical, emotional, spiritual, and social problems. Health behavior, in this instance, includes personal hygiene, dietary practices,

* Stated to J. Rash by Dr. Mohammed Allam, a former student from Egypt.

21

maintaining the sanitary environment, selection and purchase of health supplies such as patent medicines, regular dental care including visits to the dentist, selection and use of medical services, establishing and following a hygienic regimen of life, acceptable attitudes in social relationships, and a satisfactory and stabilizing spiritual experience. Perhaps it is necessary to point out that this does not imply meeting all of one's own needs alone. Indeed, this would not be an intelligent direction.

While there are degrees of health education, just as there are degrees of health, the health-educated person can recognize signs of impending illness and turn to the *proper* sources for needed assistance. At the same time such a person will be cognizant of, and practice, the living pattern that will reduce the occurrence of illness to a minimum and enhance the quality of life.

One of the most important fundamental beliefs of the health educator is that *health is related to behavior* and in many instances is dependent on it. Human beings possess enough knowledge to eradicate many, if not most, of the common killer diseases. Smallpox was reported to be eradicated from the world in 1975, through a large-scale immunization program. This was the first such accomplishment, resulting from a worldwide cooperative program under the guidance of WHO. The ultimate, and unsolved, problem is to motivate individuals to do what must be done to conserve health.

Since health is so closely related to behavior, a second fundamental belief of the health educator is that *behavior can be modified through education.* This is the ultimate role of the health educator: to strengthen the desirable and to modify the undesirable behavior patterns.

Conservation of Health

The nature of health is such that the wrong emphasis, or too much emphasis, immediately defeats the purpose. Its nature is also such that the efforts of health education should be directed at conserving health. With some notable exceptions one's quality of health is seldom better than one's potentiality for health from birth. Like a spool of thread of unknown length, it may be unwound at varying speeds. Occasionally, all too frequently, the thread is broken and life ends without playing out the maximum potential. Too often disease, stress, deprivation, dissipation, and/or such seemingly minor factors as unhygienic living, overwork, loss of sleep, etc., take their toll and, in effect, unwind the spool at an accelerated rate of speed.

Medical science is sometimes needed to assist nature in restoring the healthful condition of the organism. Health education can assist medical science by developing the intelligent self-direction of health behavior, thus conserving health and rendering it less likely that medicine be called upon to help restore health. It is important that we distinguish between health education and the practice of

22

medicine and that we understand that one of the most important contributions of health education is to promote the intelligent self-direction of health behavior to enable the individual to recognize the need for medical attention and to select and use the appropriate health services.

School Health Education

Within the school program there are two broad classifications of health education: *direct* and *indirect*. *Indirect health education*, sometimes known as incidental or sometimes as concomitant, accrues from one's everyday experiences. It is acquired by getting accustomed to clean surroundings and feeling uncomfortable when they are not clean. *Direct health education* may more properly be classified as health instruction. To expand on the definition of the Committee on Terminology, it consists of learning experiences in or through the classroom for the express purpose of favorably influencing knowledge, attitudes, and practices that will make possible the intelligent self-direction of health behavior. Health instruction may be provided effectively in health education courses (the concentrated health course) or in units or lessons in other (usually related) courses. In the latter cases the method employed may be either through direct teaching or through the method of correlation, that is, of showing the relationship of the health problem to the subject being studied (Chapter 17).

Since every teacher is, to some extent, a health teacher we might justifiably ask, "isn't every teacher an English teacher, a mathematics teacher, or a history teacher?" The answer is yes and no! Yes, to the extent that every teacher should make use of opportunities to strengthen the learnings in these areas, to correct errors, and to insist on proper use, but no in the sense that it is not possible for everyone to be responsible for everything. We have not, as yet, been able to provide sufficient educators thoroughly grounded in all aspects of knowledge (the various disciplines) to ensure the successful conduct of a completely integrated program of education. If (perhaps when) we are able to staff our schools with teachers each of whom is a composite grammarian-mathematician-scientist-historian-sociologist-health educator, at approximately the master's degree level in each area, we might assume that we have a staff capable of conducting the completely integrated program, thus making everyone a health teacher. In the meantime, except for the lower elementary grades, we would do well to direct our efforts toward providing direct health instruction plus coordination of the efforts of all who are working in areas related to health education—for example, in biology, general science, social science, physical education, and home economics, as well as health service personnel and persons concerned with maintaining the healthful environment (administrators, custodians, etc.)—at the same time stressing the need for all school personnel to see their relationships in terms of health. If this is to be accomplished, the need for an inservice health education program

23

must be recognized. Such a program should have high priority in any plans for improving the quality of the school program through inservice education.

In spite of the emphasis on health and health education, health is not an end in itself. Rather it is a means to the end of a fuller, richer, more enjoyable life that will make possible a higher service to humanity. Furthermore, it is safe to assume that health will not be conserved by making it the primary objective of life. As Hoyman indicated, "aim directly at health and you are sure to miss the target." (12:279). Important as it is, when health becomes *the* objective of life, it loses its proper place in our perspective of life and becomes like the will-o-the-wisp, always just outside one's grasp.

Concomitants from Health Instruction

Just as health education can be concomitant with other educational experiences, so are there concomitants resulting from health instruction. In terms of the objectives of education, as outlined in *Cardinal Principles of Secondary Education*, (7) health instruction is recognized as making a direct and material contribution to the objectives of health (obviously), citizenship, worthy home membership, and ethical character, and perhaps less directly to vocation, worthy use of leisure time, and command of fundamental processes. Through their practice of directing health behavior individuals may conserve and promote their own health. Through participation in community (civic) health-related activities, students are encouraged to develop a higher quality citizenship. In mastering the fundamental skills of healthful living such as care of infants, food selection and preparation, managing emotionally stressful situations, we enhance worthy home membership. And by learning that honesty is basic to dealing with one's own problems (e.g., not cheating while on a reducing diet) the foundation is laid for enlarging the scope of ethics to the larger community. However, we must not lose the perspective of the aim of health education. The concomitants are extras (for which there is no charge), and serve to enrich the total educational program.

References

1. American Association for Health, Physical Education, and Recreation, *Health Concepts: Guides for Health Instruction*, AAHPER, Washington, D.C., 1967.

2. American Association of School Administrators, *Health in Schools*, National Education Association, Washington, D.C., 1942.

3. Bauer, W.W., *Your Health Today*, Harper, New York, 1955.

4. Bobbit, Franklin, *How to Make a Curriculum*, Houghton, Chicago, 1924.

5. Beauchamp, G.A., *Curriculum Theory*, Third Edition, Kagg, Willmette, Illinois, 1975.

6. *Chronicle of the World Health Organization* 1:29–43 (1947).

7. Department of Interior, Bureau of Education, *Cardinal Principles of Secondary Education*, Bulletin No. 35, Government Printing Office, Washington, D.C., 1918.

8. Dubos, Rene, *Mirage of Health*, Anchor Books, Doubleday, Garden City, N.Y., 1959.

9. Dunn, H.L., *High-Level Wellness*, Beatty, Ltd., Arlington, Virginia, 1961.

10. Galdston, I., Editor, *Beyond the Germ Theory*, Health Education Council, New York, 1954.

11. Goodlad, J.I., R. von Stoephasius, and M.F. Klein, *The Changing School Curriculum*, The Fund for the Advancement of Education, New York, 1966.

12. Hoyman, H.S., "An Editorial: Health and a Living Faith," *The Journal of School Health*, 40:6 (1970).

13. Joint Committee on Health Problems in Education of the National Education Association and the American Medical Association, *Health Education*, Washington, D.C, 1941.

14. Salk, J., M.D., "What Do We Mean By Health?" *The Journal of School Health*, 42:10 (1972).

15. Smith, B.O., W.O. Stanley, and J.H. Shores, *Fundamentals of Curriculum Development*, Revised Edition, World, Yonkers-on-Hudson, 1957.

16. Strang, R.M. and D.F. Smiley, *The Role of the Teacher in Health Education*, Macmillan, New York, 1941.

17. Tyler, R.W., *Basic Principles of Curriculum and Instruction*, University of Chicago, Chicago, 1974, c1949.

Chapter Three
The Responsibility of the School in Health Education

The actual or real origin of the health program of the school took place with the origin of schools. From the first formally organized teaching situation, attention has been given to certain aspects of health such as physical comfort, communicable diseases, and accidents. The earliest recognition of a special school responsibility came with the realization that health and learning were interrelated. As indicated earlier, the first manifestation of this relationship was the concern for eyesight.

The potential of the school as a hotbed of infection of communicable disease was recognized in the latter part of the nineteenth century. However, the early health conservation efforts in the school health programs were directed toward the effects of health on learning. In few, if any, situations was the general welfare of the individual an important consideration.

The recent emphasis on *the whole child* and the importance of *the individual as an individual* is almost the complete antithesis of the first concerns. It is to be hoped that the emphasis on academic (intellectual) excellence does not obscure the importance of the general welfare of the individual.

Current Emphasis on Health Education

With its emphasis on the health education aspects of healthful living, health services, and health instruction, the school health education program as we know it today first began to be manifest following World War I (1918). In the face of severe criticism over the health of the inductees, as evidenced by draftees who were rejected, schools began to give special attention to the health needs of students, especially for the health education of the individual. Health instruction was first provided in regular classes, and the educational potential of health services and healthful living was recognized. In this respect schools sometimes tended to defeat their own purpose by taking over a considerable amount of the responsibility for the health problems of school children. Clinics were established in many schools and health services were provided at school expense, but too often with little or no attempt to acquaint the child with the community resources for health care that he must later depend upon as an adult. In many schools a health class was required at almost every grade level.

The currently recommended practice is to emphasize the health education opportunities in all aspects of the school program, including health instruction in related classes and/or courses, provision of special health classes or courses at designated grade levels, utilizing opportunities for health instruction in health services and healthful environment situations and wide use of community resources in meeting the health service needs.

It is a generally accepted fact that school personnel serve in the role of parents, *in loco parentis*, while the child is in school. Although this has been the accepted practice in schools in the past, conflicting ideas and ideals are serving to confuse the issue today. Three factors contribute to the need for *in loco parentis* practice: (1) someone must act in the parent role, especially for younger children, (2) the school day is becoming longer, and (3) more families have both parents working.

Factors that discourage the practice are: (1) the tendency for teachers to be less familiar with the home and the home practices of each child, because of the pressures of larger classes and the mobile population, (2) increasing independence of children, especially in the higher grade levels, and (3) implications, and implied significance, of court decisions in favor of pupils in damage suits brought against teachers. This third factor is further strengthened by some state laws prohibiting what many consider to be an essential parental responsibility for guiding and correcting behavior, and by the stress on open access to student records that discourages teachers from making essential anecdotal records regarding students.

In spite of conflicting ideas and practices, *the teacher is the substitute parent* during the school day and thus the school is the substitute home for that same period. In the role of the substitute home the school is forced to accept the corresponding responsibilities of guidance, and control if necessary.

In addition to the *in loco parentis* responsibilities the school has the primary obligation for providing an educational program. In many states this responsibility is spelled out by laws or administrative regulations concerning the time to be devoted to various subject areas, including the health area. The responsibilities for the health education program will best be carried out by encouraging *healthful living* through maintaining an environment that will promote the health and welfare of both students and staff (Chapter 14), providing *health services* that will assist in protecting and promoting the health of students and staff

(Chapter 14), and providing *health instruction* that will enable and encourage each individual to intelligently direct his or her own health behavior (Chapter 9). The sum of these experiences that favorably influence the health education of students is commonly called the *health education program*. It is important to note that this requires that there be educational experiences in each of the three phases of the program: *healthful living, health services,* and *health instruction.*

From its inception, when inspectors were first introduced into the school to detect communicable diseases and when vision tests were initiated to promote learning, the school health program has been concerned with the prevention of disease and the correction of remediable defects. As progress was made in these efforts, attention was given to education for health and longevity. In the early days of the recognized school health program, mortality rates and longevity served as excellent indices of the health of the community. With progress in the control of mortality from early childhood diseases, and the subsequent increase in life expectancy, mortality rates of school children may not now accurately reflect the true health condition of a population.

As has been pointed out by Mattison (2) and Hanlon (1:355) if mortality rates of school age children were accurate indices of health needs, there would be little need for the school health program today other than intensified accident prevention efforts. However, when morbidities, including so-called minor morbidities such as colds, carious teeth, and overweight, are used as indices, the health of school age children is seen in a different light. Furthermore, those minor morbidities may well be of increasing importance because of their possible impact on health in later years. The relationships between streptococcal infection, rheumatic fever, and possible heart impairment are well established. As a result, great importance is attached to the medical treatment of an infection that may be strep in nature, for example. The relationships of infant and childhood obesity, subclinical undernourishment, focal infections such as infected tonsils, to emotional stresses and health in later years have not been so well understood. However, these relationships are now being clarified. For example, it is generally accepted that the obese child, especially the obese infant, develops fat cells that provide the basis for adult obesity, and many psychologists now emphasize the close relationship between the love and emotional security given the infant and the personality of the adult.

In view of this situation, it is evident that the health needs of children of school and preschool age should focus on (1) providing a healthful living situation that will protect against communicable diseases, infections, and injury from accidents; (2) the correction of remediable conditions that may adversely affect health; (3) the encouragement of a diet that will maintain optimal growth and development and avoid malnutrition; (4) participation in a program of activity and rest that will promote optimal development, and fitness; (5) fostering an emotional climate that will be conducive to optimal psychological development and mental health; and (6) instruction that will provide the information, understanding, and motivation culminating in the realization of the aim of health education. All teachers and administrators should understand the relationship of these areas of need to the commonly accepted three phases of the school health program.

Some Guiding Principles for the School Health Program

To arrive at the program needed in each school, Maxwell has very appropriately suggested some guiding principles for schools of various sizes and locations:

The optimum school health program must depend upon the availability of resources, that is, resources in personnel and facilities. Both may be dependent to a large measure upon finances. (3:181)

In terms of personnel available, which is often related to the size of the school, he pointed out that the basic optimum program would provide a happy, healthful, friendly atmosphere, with:

1. A healthful and safe environment.
2. A planned and graded program of physical activities.
3. A health teaching program for health knowledge, practices, and attitudes.
4. Daily observation by the teacher.
5. An annual screening program with referrals.
6. Semiannual, or annual, visits to the dentist.
7. A school health committee (or council for a school system).

Maxwell (3) has specified additional health services and health service personnel, as the need indicates and as resources permit (Chapter 16). The healthful school environment, healthful living, is discussed in greater detail in Chapter 15 but, in connection with the school's responsibility for health education, it should be emphasized now that numerous opportunities for health education are inherent in the health service and the healthful living programs.

A healthful and safe environment is generally considered to be part of the physical environment and the emotional climate. The *healthful physical environment* is the result of a combination of conditions including safe and sanitary buildings and grounds, proper heating and ventilation, adequate lighting, proper seating, pure water and sanitary waste disposal, clean air, and a healthful and educational food service program.

The *healthful emotional climate* is dependent on such factors as the schedul-

30

ing of classes, desirable interpersonal relationships (including teacher–teacher, teacher–pupil, and pupil–pupil relationships), reasonable curricular loads for pupils and teachers, sound policies and practices in testing and marking, a satisfactory (high) level of discipline, and a democratic administration with due consideration for the total health and welfare of each individual student and staff member.

There is little doubt but that the healthful emotional climate is the direct result of an effective democratic administration. People learn to be citizens of a democratic republic by practicing that kind of citizenship and, except for the home, the school unquestionably has the greatest impact on the practices of citizenship.

In light of the need to learn adult behavior through practice in early years, it becomes essential that the school health program provide students the opportunity to acquire desirable practices, at their own level of capability, that they will use as health-educated adults. This will require, among other things, the educational approach of learning through doing in all aspects of the school program. In *healthful living* there will be opportunity: for appropriate activity, both in organized classes and in free play periods; for practicing habits of cleanliness through the use of proper facilities and supplies, hot water, soap, towels; for learning experiences through the school lunch program, whether it be the packed lunch or the food service program of the school; for putting democracy to practice in the school situation; and for learning how to live creatively, through the precept, example, and direction of a faculty that is capable of setting the desirable example.

In *health services* this means that the health needs of students and staff will be met through the kinds of practices and resources that will be used as adults. For example, since the American family looks to the family physician for medical care a planned and coordinated system of use of the private physician will be used for such health needs as examinations and immunizations as well as treatment when ill.

In *health instruction* this means a coordinated and articulated program of instruction throughout the school life of the student, with provision for correlated health teaching in related subjects and direct teaching through appropriate concentrated health courses as the needs of the students indicate. No set pattern of scheduling is recommended but schools, administration, and faculty are strongly urged to examine carefully the health education needs of the school and community and to make provision for meeting those needs.

If schools are to provide the setting in which optimum health education of the students can take place, the professional preparation of school health personnel becomes of paramount importance. Without attempting to go into detail regarding professional preparation, it seems appropriate to suggest that school administrators and school boards be aware of the kind of preparation needed by each of the professional staff—teachers, nurses, and physicians, for example—and that the professional assignments be made on the basis of total merit, including interest. This is especially true of the people who teach the health education classes.

In this connection one newer development in teacher preparation merits special consideration.

Competency Based Health Education

In recent years, the subject of competency based education has received much attention. Competency based education programs may be referred to as Competency Based Education (CBE), Competency Based Teacher Education (CBTE), Performance Based Teacher Education (PBTE), or by similar titles. Generally, CBE programs precisely specify certain behaviors to be exhibited by learners as a result of the program. In teacher education programs in particular, students must exhibit certain specified behaviors and demonstrate that children can learn as a result of the behavior.

A national study of competency based health education programs (5:15–16) provided insight into the nature and scope of these programs across the nation. A survey of more than 175 colleges and universities offering degree programs in health education produced these findings.

1. Health educators lacked consensus about what constitutes competency based health education.

2. Institutions in states where competency based education had been mandated had more elaborate competency based health education programs than institutions in other states.

3. Health educators made little use of CBE materials available from the American Association of Colleges for Teacher Education, though the AACTE has provided leadership from the beginning of the CBE movement.

4. Faculty members at the reporting institutions held widely differing views of the value of competency based education.

Various forms of competency based education exist in the country today. Some programs are concerned with professional preparation, while others involve a service activity. For example, competency based teacher education (CBTE) is a professional program concerned with producing competent teachers, but variations in programs exist within this framework. Are the teachers to be prepared for elementary or secondary school? How may the various subject areas including health education be coordinated into a total CBTE program for the elementary teacher? How may a student in a specific secondary subject matter area such as health education be included in a CBTE program? Obviously, the approach to elementary and secondary CBTE programs will be different.

In addition to professional preparation programs, some service activities such as first aid or personal health may be organized as competency based courses. In such situations, because the student is not necessarily prepared to teach others, the requirements for demonstrating competence differ from the requirements in a professional preparation program.

Based on the findings of the national study, a description of the various forms of competency based health education seems appropriate. Competency based health education programs may be categorized in six areas.

1. *Elementary Education*—In CBTE programs for the preparation of elementary teachers, a group of faculty members from various subject matter areas including Health Education cooperate as a team. The students acquire certain generic (common) teaching competencies and certain content-specific competencies specified for each of the subject areas.

2. *Secondary Education*—At the secondary level, competency based health education involves the preparation of subject matter specialists in Health Education for secondary schools. The CBTE team is composed primarily of health education faculty members. The students are expected to acquire certain generic teaching competencies, but considerable attention is devoted to acquiring content-specific competencies in Health Education.

3. *Graduate Programs*—Specifying competencies for graduate programs in health education involves both generic competencies and content-specific health education competencies. The format of such programs varies depending on whether graduate students are full or part time.

4. *Service Programs*—Health education service programs, such as first aid or personal health, normally are not concerned with developing teaching competencies due to the service nature of the program. For this reason, attention is directed toward specifying competencies to be acquired by the individual student with no attention given to the ability of the student to teach others.

5. *In-Service Education*—In-service programs in health education are concerned with health education competencies of individuals actively involved in teaching. Such programs may involve either in-service education activities or special graduate course offerings for teachers who are pursuing graduate degrees.

6. *Non-Teaching Personnel*—Competency based health education programs for non-teaching personnel involve the specification of competencies for com-

munity health educators, safety educators, school health service personnel, or others having non-teaching responsibilities in health education. In each case, the specified competencies reflect the skills necessary to perform in the area. (4:16–17)

It should be apparent that Competency Based Health Education (CBHE) may involve a service course, or it may involve a long-term effort to produce competent health education professionals. Since some health education programs involve the professional preparation of school health educators, the area should receive further consideration.

CBTE programs in Health Education should be concerned with the ability of the future teacher to promote learning among children. The essence of a CBTE program is based on this supposition: Future health educators must not only demonstrate that they have absorbed certain information, but they must demonstrate also the ability to utilize this knowledge in assisting children to improve their total health.

CBTE is neither a series of courses based on behavioral objectives nor a number of unrelated field experiences. CBTE is an organized program involving students, college faculty, principals, public school teachers, and others in a total educational program. Because a single course may be designed to achieve certain results expressed in the form of a specific behavior, such a course in itself does not represent competency based teacher education in the broadest sense. The course objectives merely prescribe the behavior to be exhibited as a result of the course. However, certain teaching competencies may require that a student complete a series of courses over an extended period of time. As a result, competency based programs must extend beyond the boundaries of individual courses.

In some programs, students and college faculty may form close relationships over several years while the student progresses through a planned sequence of learning experiences. Graduates of CBTE programs suggest that these relationships are especially valuable and meaningful to them. In planned programs, where students are actively involved with children in actual classrooms for months or years, an impressive level of professional competence can be achieved. As a result, graduates of CBTE programs feel more relaxed and at home in the classroom than do graduates of traditional teacher preparation programs. Because of their training, CBTE graduates are experienced teachers when they obtain their first teaching position. Potential employers should be impressed by this aspect of CBTE programs.

To be effective, a CBTE program must have an established philosophical base to provide a foundation for the total program and to give it direction as it develops. Institutions considering the development of a CBTE program would be wise to establish carefully a philosophical base for the program before proceeding

34

to specific program planning. The University of Georgia utilized these four basic assumptions in establishing a philosophical base for the CBTE programs operated through the College of Education.

1. Most of the competencies needed by teachers can be specified and assessed.
2. Teacher education should be field centered.
3. A teacher education program should serve as a model for effective teaching.
4. Teacher education is a joint responsibility of the public schools, the state education agency, and teacher preparation institutions. (6:3)

Before beginning the development of competency based programs in health education, college health educators should consider in detail all aspects of such an undertaking. The following questions are offered as a guide to considering the development of a CBHE program.

1. Of what value is the concept of competency based education?
2. How does the concept of competency based education affect the individuality of students enrolled in such programs?
3. How does the concept of competency based education differ in regard to professional health courses as opposed to service courses?
4. How does competency based education relate to current trends in education generally and in health education specifically?
5. What generic (common) competencies should be expected of all teachers?
6. What content-specific competencies should be required of the health educator?
7. What should be the relationship between health education competencies and a comprehensive CBTE program?
8. What are some suggestions for implementing a pilot program of competency based health education?
9. What are some potential problem areas in the implementation of a competency based health education program?
10. What are the prospects of competency based education for inservice educators and other nonteaching school health personnel?
11. What will be the impact of competency based education on current certification and accreditation practices and on health programs at professional preparation institutions?
12. How may the attainment of competencies be evaluated?

35

Once a philosophical base has been established, program planners must identify and specify the competencies to be required of the student. The University of Georgia programs identified and specified competencies through the following methods:

1. Determining needed teacher competencies by observing children to identify what children should know and do.
2. Converting existing college requirements into specific competencies to be acquired.
3. Eliciting professional and philosophical opinions from students, college faculty, and public school teachers about what constitutes effective teaching. (6)

The preceding methods allow for the active involvement of students, college faculty, and public school teachers in identifying and specifying competencies.

Generally, competencies may be classified as either *generic* (common) or *content-specific*. Generic competencies may apply to any teacher, while content-specific competencies apply to competencies in a certain subject area such as health education. For each general competency, several indicators can be identified. For each competency, one or more indicators can be selected for use in determining if the competency has been achieved.

The following example illustrates the relationship between the generic competency and the related indicators:

competency

The student determines the needs of the learner.

indicators

1. Standardized and teacher-made tests are utilized to assess the progress of the learner and the quality of instruction.
2. The learner's performance is observed and recorded.
3. The learner's performance is analyzed to determine the level of mastery.
4. The student listens and interacts with the learner to gain informal information.
5. Other indicators.

A total CBE program should include a number of carefully selected generic competencies with several related indicators. The number of indicators for each

36

competency would be determined by the feeling of CBE program personnel about how many indicators were needed to indicate attainment of the competency. There can be no one universal set of competencies and indicators because of differences in professional philosophy, the needs of particular student populations, and the nature of various subject areas.

In addition to specifying the generic competencies to be developed, health educators must develop content-specific competencies related to health education. Specification of such competencies will vary depending on whether the program involves a service course or a professional preparation curriculum. A potentially serious problem in specifying competencies results from the tendency to specify competencies that are readily measurable by an objective standard. Such a tendency poses a threat to a balanced program since objective, readily measurable competencies generally emphasize the scientific aspects of teaching, while the subjective, artistic elements of the profession are deemphasized. Unit planners often select easily measured knowledge-centered expected outcomes for the same reasons.

The specification of competencies is an essential aspect in the development of an effective CBE program. Detailed material on the development of competencies may be obtained from the agencies listed in the *Selected Sources of Information* (Appendix A). For a program to be effective, its philosophical base must be well thought out and recognizable, and competencies selected for use must accurately reflect what the program is intended to develop in the student.

Summary

Since the school provides the principal educational force in the lives of American citizens, educators cannot ignore the responsibility for the health education of the citizens of the nation. It is incumbent on health educators and school administrators to encourage the kinds of experiences that will promote intelligent self-direction of health behavior by all school personnel.

Recent trends in health education include the conceptual approach and competency-based education. The conceptual model, developed by the School Health Education Study, provides valuable guidelines for conducting a program of health education in the elementary and secondary schools. Competency based health education applies to all levels and to various kinds of health education programs. It is especially important in teacher education (CBTE).

References

1. Hanlon, J.J., *Public Health: Administration and Practice,* Mosby, St. Louis, 1974.

37

2. Mattison, B.F., M.D., "Working Together for School Health," *The Journal of School Health*, 33:4 (1963).

3. Maxwell, C.H., "An Optimum School Health Program," *The Journal of School Health*, 20:7 (1950).

4. Pigg, R.M., "Defining Competency Based Health Education," *The Eta Sigma Gamman*, 7:2 (1975). Reprinted with the permission of *The Eta Sigma Gamman*.

5. Pigg, R.M., "A National Study of Competency Based Health Education," *Health Education*, 7:4 (1976).

6. Shearron, G.F. and C.E. Johnson, *A CBTE Program in Action: University of Georgia*, Teacher Education Center, College of Education, University of Georgia, Athens, 1973.

Chapter Four
School Health Personnel: A Cooperative Approach

It is axiomatic that the school does not and cannot exist separate and apart from the rest of the community. Neither can the successful school health program operate independently of the rest of the community health program. As the late Willard W. Patty repeatedly told his students, "School health is public health in a special place."

An understanding of the relationship of the school to the rest of the community health program is basic to the concept of the cooperative approach in the school health program. Just as a close working relationship must exist between the school and the rest of the community so must such a relationship exist between all members of the school health team.

Who Makes Up the Team?

As Nemir and Schaller (1:353-375) pointed out, many persons play an important role in the conduct of the school health program. The people most closely related, or directly involved, include *administrators, teachers, pupil personnel staff* (counselors, social workers, psychologists), *nurses, physicians, dentists, custodians, bus drivers, health coordinator, food service personnel, students,* and *parents.* Although school board members also have a responsibility, this is usually exercised through the chief administrator, who acts as their agent. They have very little direct contact with the students and faculty.

In discussing the responsibilities and relationships of the members of the school health team there is a tendency to value more highly the contributions of some team members over others. Such a value judgment should be avoided since a so-called minor task of one member may be the key factor in the success of the program. Recognizing that every member of the team has an important role , let us look at some of the responsibilities of the team members.

administrators

The administrators, as representatives of the school board, contribute to the school health program through the administrative channels of budget, personnel, curricular provisions, curriculum development, inservice training programs, and their encouragement of democratic personnel relationships. By budgeting funds for supplies, equipment, and staff they provide the basics for a program. By making provisions in the curriculum for health education programs, they create the channel through which the basic essentials may function. By making provision for curriculum development projects, they ensure both the improvement of the school program and the personal growth of the people who take part in the project. By fostering democratic relationships for all school personnel, they provide the atmosphere conducive to the highest level of operation, while at the same time providing the opportunity for faculty and students to experience the goal of education for democratic living.

The true success of any administrator depends almost entirely on the cooperative approach. The administrator truly works through the other members of the team.

teachers

There are at least three classes of teachers who must share the responsibilities for health instruction in the classrooms: the full time professional health educator, the elementary school teacher, and the teacher in related areas such as physical education and biology.

Teachers make their contribution to the school health program through direct services and through their health education efforts. The contributions through direct services may consist, for example, of providing first aid when needed, observation and detection of signs of illness, conducting programs such as vision and hearing screening, and promoting healthful living through a sanitary environment and a healthful emotional climate. It is obvious that an ongoing inservice health education program is needed for teachers if they are to meet these responsibilities. The contributions through education consist of both indirect teaching, such as fostering concomitant learnings from the sanitary environment and teaching health through the correlation of health learnings with other subjects, and direct health instruction, either in health classes or in health lessons in related subjects.

As stated previously, in a very real sense every teacher is a health teacher. In most schools the teachers on the elementary school level have a full responsibility for providing instruction in health matters, often for a designated period of time each week. In addition to this direct instruction teachers can take advantage of numerous opportunities each day for incidental correlated teachings that grow out of questions asked by students or obvious relationships of health to other matters being considered. The cooperative efforts of all teachers and all pupils are essential to the effective health program.

pupil personnel staff

The contributions of members of the school staff commonly classified as pupil personnel are made in both direct services and educational efforts, chiefly through personal counseling. In much the same manner as teachers the pupil personnel staff may give first aid and observe for signs of illness. However, their best opportunities come from the personal counseling situations and the use that they make of the results of tests and other diagnostic devices and experiences. In the personal counseling situation there are countless opportunities for discussing health problems and for counseling on health attitudes and practices. Analysis of the results of diagnostic tests may give insights that can play a vital role in the health education efforts of others. It is especially important that teachers be appraised of conditions that might have an impact on their work with students. In many ways, pupil personnel staff are an important part of the team approach to solving school health problems.

nurse

The nurse is probably the most generally recognized member of the school health team. Although the routine nursing activities are important, the true value of the nurse depends on a cooperative working relationship with teachers, pupils, administrators, parents, and all others on the school health team. Working independently the nurse can, at best, only reach a few students each day. Working cooperatively the nurse can multiply his or her efforts so that every member of the school may at all times profit from these efforts.

In health services, a simple inservice education program in first aid for teachers, for example, may provide the basis for a truly successful emergency care program for a school. Advice to the administrator, and subsequently to the school board, on policies regarding excuses for illness, for both pupils and staff, may lead to vastly improved working conditions. Consultations with teachers on health instruction matters may provide the foundation for more effective teaching or a more effective coordination of teaching efforts. Health counseling of pupils and parents may lead to improved health practices, correction of

41

remediable defects, and a healthier and happier school and community. The work of the nurse is truly a cooperative effort.

physician

The physician working in the school today can best be described as a *medical educational consultant*. As Sellery (2) pointed out, the physician acts principally as a medical advisor and health consultant to the school on health problems in education. This is a far cry from the medical inspections and clinical operations of the past. The relationship of the physician to other members of the school health team is cooperative. Rarely does the medical consultant give direct service to any of the school personnel. Instead, he or she stands ready to assist in determining policies and guiding school practices that are related to the health of students and faculty. This includes assistance to teachers in planning health instruction, consultation with the administrator and the school board regarding the total school health program, and working cooperatively with the school nurse to protect and promote the health of all school personnel.

dentist or dental hygienist

The role of the dentist in the school health program, like that of the physician, is generally as a dental educational consultant. Only in rare instances does a dentist actually practice dentistry in the school. Most dental care that is provided in the school is the work of the dental hygienist. Even in these cases the work is usually limited to prophylaxis, with an emphasis on getting students under regular preventive dental care. The most significant contribution of the dentist or dental hygienist is to serve as a resource and consultant on dental problems, so that students actually carry out good dental health practices of hygiene, nutrition, and dental care. Such assistance includes working with teachers in planning good instruction in dental care, consultation with the administration regarding the school dental health program, and working cooperatively with the school nurse to protect and promote dental health of all school personnel.

custodian

The custodian can make a significant contribution to the school health program as a member of the school health team. The work of the custodian has both a direct and an educational influence on the health of all school personnel. In helping to maintain the healthful environment, the custodian directly contributes to the health of the students and staff by helping to protect them from possible infections, irritations (emotional and physical), and accident hazards. Custodians provide an atmosphere for concomitant learnings. Students who become accustomed to a clean, pleasant, and safe environment learn to desire that kind of environment and are dissatisfied with anything less agreeable. When teachers cooperate with custodians by using the healthful environment as a teaching device, the educational contribution of the custodian is enhanced. The cooperative efforts of all school personnel are required, and such efforts tend to encourage further and more effective cooperation.

bus driver

In schools where transportation is provided bus drivers can play an important role in health conservation and health education. In addition to ensuring a safe, healthful, and pleasant mode of transportation, they can make early identification of the signs of communicable disease and, thus, prevent their widespread exposure on the bus and in school. They are also in position to make astute observations of pupil behavior such as evidence of abuse in the home or unusually belligerent behavior. By reporting these observations to the proper authorities, the bus drivers can enhance the work of the school health team.

In some instances, the bus driver can be a confidant and friend of students who may lack such a relationship, such as the fatherless boy. It is, indeed, important that the bus drivers be consciously included on the school health team.

food services personnel

The school lunch program has the potential for being one of the most effective instructional systems in the school. This potential can only be realized through the cooperative working relationship of the food service personnel, the health education personnel, and the administrators. If health education, including nutrition education, is to result from the experiences associated with the school lunch program, there must be planned cooperation to that end.

The food service personnel can contribute both to health protection through exemplary food handling and preparation and to health education through participation in planning and conducting a nutrition education program of all school personnel. The health education aspect, especially, requires the cooperative effort of administrators, food service personnel, teachers, and students.

health coordinator

The health coordinator is *the key person* on the school health team, the one whose entire efforts are devoted to promoting the cooperative approach. Except in instances where the size of the school does not justify a full-time position for the coordinator, that person will devote full-time to facilitating, expediting, and motivating the cooperative and coordinated efforts of all school personnel. In schools where the coordinator has teaching responsibilities, that portion of time allowed for the coordination responsibilities will be used in this way. The promotion of inservice education is one of the important responsibilities of the coordinator.

The position of the coordinator is unique in that it is an arm of administration but it is without administrative authority. It cannot be compared with the supervisor because the supervisor is primarily concerned with the instruction curriculum, with well-defined administrative responsibility, while the health coordinator is concerned with the attitudes and practices of all school personnel in all areas of the school health program including the healthful environment, health services, and health instruction. Furthermore, the very nature of the job dictates that it be a position without authority. It should be well understood that people cannot be forced to work together in a friendly cooperative manner. If the coordinator has to have authority to force coordination, it defeats the purpose while if the purpose is achieved, if only partially, the authority is not needed. The success of the coordinator is indicated by the degree to which coordination of the efforts of the school health personnel is achieved without the exercise of authority.

The responsibilities, or opportunities, of the coordinator include:

1. Planning ways to create a closer working relationship between teachers and the health service and custodial personnel.

2. Encouraging all teachers to inform others of their plans for health teaching and to find out what is being taught by other teachers.

3. Participating in and encouraging curriculum planning for health education and helping develop long range plans for health instruction, a course of study, to ensure that important points not be neglected and that there not be needless repetition between related teachings (e.g., biology and health) or from year to year (e.g., repetition in high school of what is taught in the lower grades).

4. Promoting the use of community resources and facilities in the health instruction program and aiding in such use by making appropriate contacts and assisting in scheduling speakers, planning field trips, and keeping teachers informed of developments in the community.

5. Providing essential instructional materials, screening new publications and new materials, and making appropriate ones available to members of the school health team.

6. Fostering interpersonal relationships to promote a closer working relationship of all members of the school health team.

Coordination is a key to an effective total school health education program. Development of the program through the cooperative procedures suggested provides the foundation for the effective working together of all school personnel, which is essential. However, it does not guarantee such a relationship. Effective coordination of effort results from planned, deliberate, attempts to involve people in the work they can do most effectively. It rarely happens by chance.

Even though the coordinated program is brought about by planning, this will not ordinarily be apparent to the casual observer. In fact, it may not be readily apparent to those involved, including the administrator to whom the coordinator is responsible. The most effective coordination is brought about when the people who are most directly involved often do not realize that their actions have been influenced by a third party. It has been pointed out that when the work of the coordinator is truly successful, the people will feel that *we did it ourselves.*

students

The students in a school play a dual role in the health program. They are both the recipients and the participants. It is sufficient to mention that the benefits to pupils from the optimum school health program include the protection of their health, promotion of a higher quality health, encouragement and assistance when needed for correction of remediable defects, help in learning to live successfully with defects that cannot be corrected, and the opportunity for decision making regarding their own health behavior. The role of students as participants in achieving these benefits includes active and willing participation in all aspects of the program including individual responsibilities in the daily health observation program, first aid preparation, teamwork in screening programs, sincere participation in the instructional program including conscious efforts to use the desirable practices that are taught, wise use of community health services as they may be needed from time to time, and communication of their needs to the proper persons.

Success in the school health program hinges as much if not more on the cooperative efforts of students as on any other members of the school. The students may very well be the final authority in the success of the school health program. It is they who consider, choose, or discard, and practice or not practice the health conservation measures that are being encouraged.

parents

Just as the school situation dictates that teachers act *in loco parentis*, so does the home situation dictate that parents act as teachers. The teaching responsibilities of the parents are so numerous and significant as to be almost overwhelming. It is a well-established fact that children come to school with ideas and emotional sets so firmly established that it is difficult and, in some cases, impossible to change them. Fortunately for all concerned, but especially for the students, the normal home situation provides the setting for desirable learnings. The role of the parents in the school health program is consciously to foster such an environment and by so doing to reinforce the efforts of the school.

If parents are to reinforce the efforts of the school, it should be obvious that clear channels of communication and close cooperation must exist. There must be a free, two-way, flow of information. Parents must understand and support the goals and efforts of the school. They must know what teachers want and expect, and they need to be informed of both the success and failures of the students in carrying out the teachings in all aspects of living. In a like manner teachers must know something of the expectations and the goals of parents. These can only be ascertained through personal contact with the parents. Little can be accomplished, especially in modifying undesirable health behavior, when teachers and parents are working at cross purposes. It must be a cooperative effort.

The importance of a cooperative working relationship between all members of the school health team is so crucial that some mechanism for implementing it must be provided. One of the approaches for achieving this cooperation is through the school health council and committee system (Chapter 6). The school health council can provide the medium for coordination between schools within a school system, and the school health committee can serve the same function in the individual school. At the community level a community health council can serve as a coordinating agency for community-wide programs involving different agencies.

Summary

No other aspect of the total school program relies as much on the success of the cooperative efforts of all members of the school team as does the school health program. Some of the cooperation may occur incidentally in the normal course of the school program, but the incidental too often turns out to be accidental. *A truly cooperative effort* must be planned and carried out in a systematic manner, and the role of the coordinator is vital to the success of such efforts.

The responsibilities of all members of the school health team should be clearly defined and arrived at in a democratic manner. If it is the responsibility of the school to teach people to live in a democratic society under a republican form of government, then the school has the inescapable responsibility of providing the opportunity for developing the desired attitudes and practices to be used in our democratic society.

References

1. Nemir, A. and W.E. Schaller, *The School Health Program*, Saunders, Philadelphia, 1975.
2. Sellery, E.M., "Where Are We Going in School Health Education," *The Journal of School Health*, 20:151–159 (1950).

46

Chapter Five
Community Resources for Health Education

When the school health program is viewed as an integral part of the total community health program, which is its true relationship, it becomes clear that the school must *both serve and depend on the community*. Just as any branch of government or any other community institution has its own special prerogatives, procedures, and responsibilities, the school is an institution with a special responsibility and, therefore, a unique program. However, only as this unique program functions, cooperatively, as a member of the whole community program, making its unique contribution, can the total program approach its optimum effectiveness.

If the students who attend our schools are to be able to direct their own health behavior in an intelligent manner, then use of community resources for health is one of the health practices that must be encouraged. This practice can and must be nurtured by the school, and the most effective teaching in this regard is the use of (or association with) community resources throughout the school life of the individual. Learning, especially the development of desirable attitudes and practices, is most effective when actual practice is involved. We learn by doing and, if that learning is to be desirable, it is imperative that proper guidance be given at appropriate times.

Since education for citizenship is a recognized goal of our schools, it follows that the highest level of citizenship involves understanding, using, and supporting the worthy programs and institutions of the community. To the extent that the school health program contributes to the understanding, use, and support of all aspects of the community health program, it will also contribute to attaining the goal of citizenship.

47

Community Resources

To be able to work cooperatively with the resources of the community, teachers must know what resources are available and understand their functions and responsibilities in the community program. Such resources may exist outside the immediate geographical community and still be available. In this respect, community resources may be said to be both *local* and *state* (sometimes even national or international).

There are at least six common classifications of community resources, or agencies, that participate in the school health education program. These are the (1) official agencies, (2) voluntary agencies (including foundations), (3) professional associations, (4) sponsored agencies, (5) civic (or service) clubs, and (6) consumer services. Some of these resource agencies are shown by classification in Figure 2.

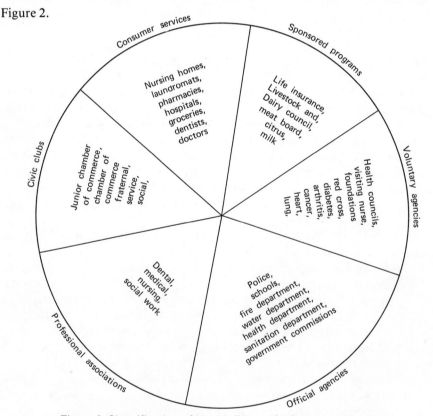

Figure 2. Classification of Health Education Resources for the School Health Education Program.

48

The most productive learning experiences involve the direct use of or participation in the service or activity. As Dale (1) pointed out, direct participation provides the best learning situation while verbalization is usually least effective.

As the learning experiences of the student involve less and less direct participation, their effectiveness diminishes, much as the surface area of a cone or triangle decreases with each successive step away from the base (representing direct participation). This relationship of participation to learning is important because it is the basis for the need to involve students in the actual practice of community living if they are to learn to participate in community life. When direct participation is not possible the effective teacher resorts to other, less direct, methods, but the emphasis is on that procedure or method that most closely simulates actual community living. To this end, student organizations such as the student council, and student voluntary health agencies such as the Red Cross or the Heart Association become effective substitutes for actual participation in the adult version of the same activity.

Now let us examine, briefly, the various community resources for health education.

official agencies

In most countries of the world the health department, or the ministry of health, has the official responsibility for safeguarding and promoting the health of the people. It is significant that the governmental, tax-supported, agency we call the health department is so nearly uniform in structure worldwide. Various international organizations, including the League of Nations and the World Health Organization, have contributed to the worldwide pattern of the health department.

In the United States of America the local health department carries the main responsibility for health protection and promotion. The local health department may be part time or full time, and it may be a city, county, city-county, or multiple county health department.

In addition to the health department, other official agencies, sometimes called public agencies, are responsible for certain aspects of health and safety; these include the police department, the fire department, schools, and certain departments of government such as the water and sanitation departments. In general, it may be said that an official public health agency is any *tax-supported agency having responsibility for health.*

Final authority in health matters may rest either with the local board of health or the state health department, depending on state laws, but such authority is ordinarily exercised through the local department. State health departments in turn, look to the Public Health Service of the U.S. Department of Health, Education and Welfare for consultation, guidance, and support in matters that affect

49

the health of our citizens. In general, the authority of Public Health Service is limited to matters of *interstate concern*, but the state health departments look to and are guided by the federal health agency in a spirit of cooperation. On the international level the federal agencies of the member countries look to the World Health Organization for counsel and guidance in the public health program.

In the past, schools (or teachers) have been remiss in not calling on and working with the health department of their community and state. Since our present pattern of health department organization started with the passage of the Social Security Act, in 1935, in terms of the history of education it is a young agency. As school people become better acquainted with the health department they may make better use of its resources.

Since it is a recognized responsibility of schools to educate our citizens on citizenship, such educational activities should take advantage of the resources of the official health agency. It is significant that the health department has the support of the other health agencies, including professional and voluntary agencies. It should be a goal of every school that every student should *understand, use*, and *support the local health department.* Methods of doing this are considered in Chapter 16, but the most effective educational procedure to accomplish this goal is *actual participation.*

voluntary agencies

The voluntary health agency, sometimes referred to as the private agency, is distinctly a North American (U.S.A.) phenomenon. Although to a limited extent it has spread to other parts of the world, it had its origin in the United States of America with the development of voluntary nursing services and with the organization of the Anti-Tuberculosis Society of Philadelphia in 1892 and the National Association for the Study and Prevention of Tuberculosis in 1904. (2:309) Other voluntary health agencies soon began to appear and today there is hardly a disease or disorder that is not represented by its corresponding *Association.*

Although voluntary agencies are often classified into four classes (2:311), five classes are suggested here. These are the agencies concerned with: (1) *a specific disease*: cancer, muscular dystrophy, myasthenia gravis; (2) *certain organs or structures*: heart, lung, kidney; (3) *health and welfare of special groups*: maternity, child health, the crippled; (4) *a particular phase of health and welfare*: safety, sanitation, emergencies (Red Cross); and (5) foundations.

While foundations such as the Rockefeller Foundation, the W.K. Kellogg Foundation, the Carnegie Foundation, and the Russell Sage Foundation are supported by voluntary contributions, they fall into a rather special classification because they do not ordinarily ask the general public for support. For this reason we think of them as falling into a fifth classification of voluntary agencies. They are most often established by an individual or a family. They are, as are the other voluntary agencies, distinctly a North American (and capitalistic) phenomenon having their origin in the desire of some wealthy individuals to give money to worthy causes and to enjoy certain tax reduction benefits in so doing.

In contrast with the *official*, tax-supported, health agency the *voluntary health agency is supported by voluntary contributions*. In view of their specialized interests and flexibility of programs the voluntary agencies are meeting a very definite need today. In general they supplement, rather than duplicate or supplant, the services of the official agencies. In many instances they are able to pioneer and to meet health needs that the official agency may not be permitted to do.

Since the voluntary agencies constitute an important part of the public health program of our communities, it is vitally important that our citizens be taught to understand, use, and intelligently support these agencies.

professional associations

One of the chief goals of professional associations in a community is to foster greater unity among their members. However, professional associations are also dedicated to improving the quality of professional preparation and service and one of the ways this can be done is by increasing an understanding in the community of what its members do.

Professions that ordinarily have local associations include physicians (local medical society), dentists (constituent dental societies), nurses (local nurses' association or club), and teachers. Public health employees, veterinarians, optometrists, social workers, and various governmental employees are some of the professional groups having regional or state associations.

In the past many educators, including administrators, have not worked closely with the professional associations in their communities. Full advantage should be taken of the opportunity to get physician and dentist input into curriculum development projects. School health personnel should develop regular lines of communication with other health professionals to discuss health problems occurring within the school. These local or regional professional groups can provide counsel and guidance and, in some instances, direct services to schools, *when requested*. In Indiana, for example, both the state medical and the state dental associations have gone on record, urging their members to provide counsel and guidance to school administrators and teachers, *on request*. However, school personnel must initiate the action. Other professional personnel hesitate to take the initiative because they do not want to seem to infringe on the rights of others to manage their own affairs.

sponsored agencies

Industries and businesses have long been interested in certain aspects of the health education of consumers. Sometimes the interest is not without its mercenary aspects, but in *most instances* such efforts are remarkably free of a direct advertising appeal.

Life insurance companies were probably the first business to carry on actively health education activities. In recent years numerous manufacturers, producers, and/or food processors have developed educational programs. In most instances the educational program is a corollary or supplementary program, often under a department of the sponsoring business or industry. For example, the Metropolitan Life Insurance Company has conducted an extensive educational program, the meat producers support such a program through the National Livestock and Meat Board, and the dairy interests are represented in the field of education through the National Dairy Council.

For some time the term "commercial agency" was used to identify these agencies. However, the word "commercial" gave an erroneous impression of the purpose of the agency. The term "sponsored agency"was coined and applied to an educational program that is sponsored, and usually financed, by a business or industry. Often the name of the sponsored agency does not identify the sponsoring agency, but the vested interests, if any, are usually apparent, and it is generally agreed that the educator should know what interests are represented or promoted through such a program.

Numerous educational materials are available free of charge from sponsored agencies. These include resource documents and materials, publications of current interest, sample materials, and suggestions of the sponsoring agency. Since these constitute a valuable resource for the busy teacher, the health-educated citizen must certainly be aware of them.

civic (service, social, and fraternal) clubs

Almost all communities large enough to be called cities have a variety of civic, service, social, or fraternal clubs. Many of the service clubs have programs with health implications. The sight conservation committee and the health and welfare committee of the Lions Club are examples of such a health program. Kiwanis, Optimists, Exchange, and Rotary clubs are some of the other men's service clubs that have committees with a health and safety responsibility. Some social clubs, such as the Elks and Moose, have similar programs. Such activities for women are often channeled through service sororities, church organizations, and such organizations as the Junior League, and League of Women Voters.

The civic clubs constitute a valuable resource for health activities. Their contribution is probably most often made by providing needed help in securing health service, such as glasses, or in providing support for specialized programs such as camping. These make it possible to insure more nearly equal opportunity for all, regardless of the financial situation of the parents.

consumer services

It may seem somewhat unusual to consider consumer services as a health education resource, but every community has a variety of services that can serve the purposes of health education.

The consumer services of the typical middle-size or large community are so numerous that it would be difficult to list them all. Physicians, nurses, and dentists are represented by the corresponding professional associations, but their direct services are provided by individuals. Community services such as hospitals, nursing homes, drug stores, laundries, and the many other retail stores handling products have a direct relationship to health needs. In many instances these services will have a negative influence on health education unless definite plans are made to make them a positive influence. For example, in the drug store the wise or unwise sale and use of nonprescription medicines can depend, in part, on the cooperative efforts of school and community health educators and pharmacists.

When the consumer services of a community are related to community health needs, it becomes obvious that *consumer education* is one of the most important responsibilities of the school. If students are to use intelligently the vast complex of health-related services of a community, they must learn about them early in their education and have constant exposure to them. Furthermore, each of the consumer services of the community can make its unique contribution to the educational process, provided proper plans are made and carried out by the students and teacher.

some recent developments

The material support of school health education programs by the federal government has been notably absent. Not until the mid-nineteen seventies did the federal government make any apparent concentrated effort to support school health education. The movement to support health education efforts was manifest in the establishment of the Bureau of Health Education in the Public Health Service of the Department of Health, Education and Welfare. Located in the Center For Disease Control, Atlanta, Georgia, the Bureau provides services to both school and public health educators. For example, the Bureau provides leadership and financial support for the Elementary School Health Education Curriculum Project (Chapter 10). The monthly publication, *Focal Points*, can be a valuable resource for teachers.

About the same time that the Bureau of Health Education was moved to Atlanta, the National Center for Health Education was established. The Center for Health Education is a nongovernmental (voluntary) agency, located in San Francisco, California. It serves as a national focal point within the private sector to promote the coordination and upgrading of health education efforts. Hopefully, school programs will receive equal attention and support along with public health education.

In recent years, increasing legislative attention has been directed toward the promotion of health education. Two laws, enacted during the mid-1970s, had a significant influence on the development of school and community health education programs.

Public Law 93-641, the National Health Planning and Resources Development Act of 1974, (3,4) was enacted in response to the unmistaken need for more effective coordination and the utilization of existing health resources at local, state, and federal levels. Likewise, the measure established a much-needed framework to promote effective future planning for health care facilities, health services, and health personnel. To accomplish the task, an allocation of $1,000,000,000 dollars was provided to support the measure for an initial three-year period.

Title XV of the measure had direct implications for health education. Among other stipulations, the regulation instructed the Secretary of the Department of Health, Education and Welfare to create a National Council on Health Planning and Development. Significantly, a specific responsibility of the Council was to develop procedures for instructing the public in the areas of personal health promotion and the selection and utilization of health services.

In addition to the preceding stipulation, Title XV of the measure established a national system for developing health resources and for coordinating health planning activities. Coordinating bodies were established at the state level, and a network of individual Health System Agencies was created to meet the particular needs of specific regions within each state. Since the regional HSA's responsibilities included planning for health education, some health educators found the HSA to be a positive source of support for local health education activities.

Public Law 94-317, the National Consumer Health Information and Health Promotion Act of 1976, (5,6) marked a significant legislative advancement of the cause of health education. All three titles of the legislation contributed in some way to the promotion of health education. However, the greatest support for health education resulted from Title I, "Health Information and Health Promotion."

The Secretary of the Department of Health, Education and Welfare was authorized to implement the legislation. Though detailed responsibilities were delineated, the regulation instructed the Secretary to assume general responsibility for:

1. Establishing national goals related to the effective use of health information to promote personal health and the effective utilization of health services.

2. Identifying current and projected resource requirements for the effective implementation of the national goals.

3. Initiating and supporting projects related to the national goals of encouraging the effective utilization of health information and services by the public.

4. Promoting and assisting in the exchange of material concerning health information and the promotion of personal health.

Specific responsibility for the implementation of the proposed programs was accomplished through the establishment of the Office of Health Information and Health Promotion. General responsibilities of the Office included:

1. Support of research projects designed to determine the nature and effectiveness of various health education programs.

2. Initiation and encouragement of the development of community health programs in schools and in public and private community health facilities.

3. Support of the dissemination of information concerning personal health promotion and the effective utilization of community health services.

In addition to the preceding general responsibilities, the Office was instructed to establish a national clearinghouse for health information. The purpose of the clearinghouse was to improve the availability of information related to health, health education, personal health promotion, and the utilization of health services. Emphasis was also placed on the importance of correlating activities of the Office with similar projects sponsored by nongovernmental sources.

Though Title I of PL 94-317 dealt extensively with health education and information, Titles II and III of the law also had implications for health education. Support for school health education programs was specifically included in the titles. Health education was cited as an effective element in the control and prevention of disease, with venereal disease and lead poisoning receiving particular attention.

PL 93-641 and PL 94-317 gave significant legislative support to the cause of health education. With the enactment of the laws, needed attention was focused on health education as a distinct discipline, and governmental support for health education was forthcoming. As a result, health educators were provided with the opportunity and resources to engage in meaningful program planning, implementation, and evaluation.

The impact of these movements on school health education programs will be indirect, but health educators have the responsibility to acquaint their students

55

with all aspects of health and health care, including the health service delivery systems and alternatives within those systems. The future holds much that cannot be predicted, both in quality and cost of health care. While the health educator is committed to the conservation of health, to the end that illness be eliminated or reduced to a minimum, provision must also be made for the intelligent self-direction in the use of needed health services.

Summary

The school is the principal formal educational agency in the United States of America. If our historic capitalistic-democratic way of life is to be preserved, the school must carry the main burden of preserving it. This responsibility can *only* be carried out effectively if schools follow the best principles of education and *involve the students in the kind of living they are being educated to preserve.*

It is an accepted principle that we learn to do by doing. If our citizens are to *understand, use,* and *support* the *community health resources*, they must have the opportunity to use them. Contrary to some thinking, this does not place an intolerable additional burden on the classroom teacher. Rather it opens up vast new resources (community health resources) that can be brought into action for the education of our citizens in our accepted way of life.

References

1. Dale, E., *Audio-Visual Methods in Teaching*, Dryden, New York, 1954.
2. Hanlon, J.J., *Principles of Public Health Administration*, Mosby, St. Louis, 1974.
3. 93rd U.S. Congress, Public Law 93-641, "National Health Planning and Resource Development Act of 1974," U.S. Government Printing Office, Washington, D.C., 1974.
4. Rubel, E.J., "Implementing the National Health Planning and Resources Development Act of 1974," *Public Health Reports*, 91:3-8 (January-February, 1976), in "Health Planning—A Special Section."
5. 94th U.S. Congress, Public Law 94-317, "National Consumer Health Information and Health Promotion Act of 1976," U.S. Government Printing Office, Washington, D.C., 1976.
6. "Public Law 94-317: Title I," *Focal Points*, Bureau of Health Education, (CDC-PHS-DHEW), September, 1976.

Chapter Six
The School in the Community Health Program

Growth and development, as we know it in the human organism, is not without its growing pains. The profession of health education is a young and growing profession and as such it is subject to many trials, tribulations, and traumatic experiences, much as are growing human organisms.

One of the growing pains of our profession has been a cleavage between school health and public health education. This cleavage has resulted in two widely divergent points of view concerning the work of the health educator. The school view holds that the health educator is a teacher while in the public health point of view the health educator is a community organizer, doing little if any actual teaching. It is our purpose to consider how the rather specialized areas of school health and public health can be brought into a closer working relationship.

Recognizing that there are large areas of agreement, we also know that there is often a lack of understanding. There are places where a close working relationship has been established but, since there are many places where this is not true, let us look at the needs for such action. We shall then turn our attention, in succession, to the unique features of each program, their common elements, and to some ways in which the gap between them may be bridged.

In this consideration we are primarily concerned with the educational aspects of these programs. It is generally accepted that the success of any school or public health program depends on the extent to which it is conducted as an educational program.

School health work had its beginning as a responsibility of health workers outside the school. As the program grew, and as the education profession developed, the school gradually assumed more responsibility. The history of the ad-

* This chapter is based on an article by Rash that was published in *The Journal of School Health* under tht title of "Bridging the Gap Between School Health and Public Health," *30*, 1, (1960). Used with the permission of the American School Health Association.

57

ministration of the health service program in schools reveals this pattern very clearly. From the early control of school health services by the public health department we moved to a program largely administered by school people. A third pattern has been developed in recent years, that of joint administration. This may well represent a basic link between school health and public health.

The nature of the administration of the health service program represents one of the major problem areas in school health. At the same time, within the school health service program we find that the difference in philosophy of whether nurses are employed by the school or employed by the health department represents another, somewhat more focal, point of disagreement if not real conflict.

In health education, the gap between the school health educator and the community health educator was mentioned rather prominently, and pointedly, in the 1948 report of "Educational Qualifications of Community Health Educators" (3) when the committee specifically delimited its consideration to public health educators, excluding the school health educators. At about that same time a new professional association, The Society for Public Health Educators, subsequently changed to the Society for Public Health Education, was organized for the express purpose of providing a meeting ground for persons engaged in public health education. One of the primary concerns of the Society for Public Health Education, SOPHE, has been the standards of professional preparation of health education specialists. A Task Force, chaired by Helen S. Ross, submitted to SOPHE "Guidelines for the Preparation and Practice of Professional Health Educators." (10) As indicated by the title, those guidelines focused on the health educator as a community worker, not on the school health educator.

The 1949 reorganization plan for the American Association for Health, Physical Education, and Recreation included a section on Community Health Education. The American School Health Association opened its membership to persons outside of school health service in 1937, while the American College Health Association began admitting to membership those from outside health service in the fall of 1958. Suffice it to say, we have been slow in developing or establishing satisfactory lines of communication within our own professional groups.

If we are going to increase interagency cooperation, it may be helpful to compare the two programs. In what ways do the school health program and the public health program differ, in what ways are they alike, and what are some things that may be done to promote a closer working relationship?

Features Unique to School Health Education

The school program is a *required program*. Legal requirements make it mandatory that a school be operated following a rather rigidly prescribed pattern. While legislation regarding health instruction is not universal, Castile and Jerrick

(2) reported, in 1976, that 33 states certified teachers in health education, and 16 states mandated comprehensive health education, while certification in special areas was so widespread that it left only three states with no provision at the state level for health education certification. This has led to a fairly uniform curriculum with subsequent certification regulations. In general the school has been, and is now, *knowledge centered*, and some would have it even more so.

The very nature of the school program tends to make *the teacher an authority*, both in subject and in situation. The teacher who is not able to answer students' questions or to assist them in finding the answers will not be consulted by the students. The teacher does not have on immediate call a staff of, for example, engineers, nurses, physicians, and dentists who can be called into the classroom on short notice. Furthermore, it is not feasible that they be called into the classroom regularly. Imagine the demands on the community health department if the teachers of a particular health jurisdiction began calling for members of the health department to come to the classroom every time a health problem arose.

In a community of 50,000 people (a small health jurisdiction) there are about 10,000 students in school (K–12). Divide these into classes of 25, with a teacher for every 6 classes and you have some 67 teachers, meeting 400 classes per day. Although all of these classes are not dealing with health problems every day, there could be an impossible demand on the health department if the teachers did not have basic knowledge. It is necessary that the teacher be an authority on some things other than method. This is not to imply that members of the health department should not be called into the classroom. They should be called upon as resource persons, but not to do the teaching.

One survey (6) contacting approximately 100 teachers found that teachers did not seem to encounter questions on problems in areas where they had limited preparation. It was concluded that students soon learn where they can get the answers and they go there for them. Thus, it behooves teachers to be well informed on health matters, including community resources.

Another unique feature of the school is that of *academic marks*. Testing and evaluation play such an important part in marking that it is imperative that the teacher be skilled in test construction and in evaluating test results (Chapter 20.) This necessity for marking, with the need for tests and other evaluation procedures, may constitute one of the greatest differences between the school health program and the public health program. Evaluation is an important aspect of public health programs, but such evaluation does not include the necessity for determining academic marks.

Perhaps the two most unique features of the school are that it presents a *captive audience* and that this audience is a fairly *homogeneous group*. It is a safe assumption that the graded classroom presents a more homogeneous audience than is to be found in consumers of mass media such as newspapers, radio, television, or even mass meetings.

Academic freedom of teachers constitutes another of the unique features of the school, and not the least significant in creating the gap. This operates most effectively at the teacher education level, giving a supply of teachers reflecting a wide variety of philosophy, knowledge, and methods. For teachers this freedom extends to the selection of the subject matter to be included in the classroom. Within broad limits teachers are free to choose what they teach. This is a far different situation from the food handlers course in which strict standards must be taught.

Features, such as the following, tend to make the school program unique: (1) it is a required program, (2) it is knowledge centered, (3) the teacher is an authority, (4) academic marks are necessary, (5) there is a captive audience, (6) there are homogeneous groups, and (7) there is academic freedom.

Features Unique to Public Health Education

In considering the features unique to public health there is a temptation to think only of the converse of those features unique to school health. However, it is desirable to be more specific if possible.

The first unique feature is that the public health program is commonly a *permissive program* rather than a required one. Within rather broad limits the nature of the public health program is commonly determined at the local level. A part-time health department is still legal in some places. Furthermore, the control exercised by the state health department differs considerably from that exercised by the department of public instruction that determines curriculum, sets standards for attendance, certifies teachers, and provides money to pay the base salary of a high proportion of the school staff. The state health department, in turn, is more concerned with technical standards such as air pollution, sanitation, and safety. There is little in the health department standards comparable to the regulations governing days of school, attendance laws, and curriculum requirements of the department of public instruction.

The *availability of authorities* constitutes a unique feature of the public health program. The nature of the organization of the health department leads to making the professional personnel authorities in their own fields, leaving the health educator to be an authority in method, not in subject matter. If there is need for medical knowledge the health educator is expected to turn to the physician; for dental knowledge, to the dentist; in sanitation, to the sanitary engineer, etc. This is probably one of the most unique features of the public health program.

It is also important that *the entire public health program be health centered.* In addition to having a staff of highly skilled specialists on hand, the availability of specialists in certain aspects of health creates a unique situation. The thinking and action of this staff of health experts can be, and is, directed toward the single goal, or consideration, of health.

Almost complete *freedom from a prescribed curriculum* is one of the more distinctive characteristics of the public health program. Of course, there are requirements that have to be met, but there is nothing that serves to stereotype the program to the extent that state imposed requirements for graduation do to the school program. Furthermore (and fortunately) lawmakers, lobbyists, and others who influence legislation may be a little more inclined to leave the making of health regulations to the experts than is the case with school regulations. Legislators feel free and obligated to enact laws requiring certain courses. After all, everyone is an expert in school matters. Almost everyone who is in a position to have his influence felt has spent 16 or more years in school and that just about qualifies him on school problems. Fortunately, the health department is fairly free of this problem.

Because the public health program is largely *community centered*, rather than centered in the building housing the staff, it is set off rather sharply from the school program.

Granted that the school program need not be confined to the building, it still must be centered there, whereas the public health program continues to operate, and sometimes quite well, even in the absence of a headquarters building. The better part-time departments have illustrated this feature.

Thinking specifically of the health education program, the health educator in the public health program must rely on mass media to a very great extent. Mass media do not seem to be very effective in changing behavior, at least their effectiveness has not been clearly established. Since studies in the field of social psychology do substantitate the theory that personal influence is the most effective force in securing a change in behavior, the next step is to discover how personal influence can be brought to focus on community health problems. This may be another of the gaps. Perhaps the school situation gives teachers an advantage in this case, because of the natural close personal contact of teacher and pupils. In any event, we might say the use of *mass media* is a characteristic of the public health education program. The absence of the captive audience that characterizes the school may help account for this difference, but it still has to be considered.

The features, then, that tend to make the public health program unique include: (1) it is a permissive program, (2) authorities are available, (3) it is health centered, (4) there is freedom from prescribed curriculum, (5) it is community centered, and (6) mass media are in common use.

Elements Common to School Health and Public Health Education

The first, and perhaps the foremost, element common to these programs is the *educational nature* of the program. Fundamentally, each program must be educational. It is contended that unless a program, or activity, is basically educational it has no place in the school program. We might not go quite this far in the public

61

health field, but there is general agreement that people must be helped to help themselves. After we have done *for* people whatever we must do *for* them, then the main emphasis must be on teaching them to do for themselves. Here, the goal of intelligent self-direction is especially appropriate.

The second common element is that *both programs are health programs.* In fact, both programs are public health programs. It is a matter of very great concern that the school program is so commonly set apart as something different and separate from the public health program.

A third common element is that *both programs are community programs.* They are both concerned with protection and promotion of community health, working in and through a recognized community agency. Both might be said to be dedicated to preserving the cultural values of the community.

The fourth common element is that school health and public health are *both concerned with human welfare.* We have come a long way from the early concepts of the school health program of merely making it possible to train the mind. From the concept of preventing disease or defect in order that students could learn, we have come to the place where we are concerned over disease and defect because of their impact on the total individual. We are concerned with the individual because that person is sacred and worthy of the good things in life, not just because we want information or skills in the training of the mind.

The features, then, common to the school and the public health programs include: (1) both are educational in nature, (2) both are health programs, (3) both are community programs, and (4) both are concerned with human welfare.

Bridging the Gap

If, as has been suggested, there are basic differences as well as prominent common elements, how can we bridge the gap that does exist?

First, we must recognize that the gap is wider in some communities than in others. Indeed, in some there may be no gap while in others there may be a gap, but durable and serviceable bridges may have been built.

Imagine a picture of a community in which there is a gap. On the one side you have public health that may be pictured as having the different divisions, or services, of the health department. These include the administration, public health nursing, sanitation, nutrition, preventive medicine, maternal and child health, laboratory, and education.

On the opposite side of the gap we have the school health program, made up of administration, school nursing, environmental sanitation (custodians), nutrition, preventive medicine (doctors and dentists), child welfare services (counselors, school workers, etc.), and health education (including safety education and physical education). What does it take to bridge the gap, and once we have the bridge how can we get people to use it?

The building materials for such a bridge may be found in councils, committees, and key individuals, and these are commonly inherent in the community. What is needed in most cases is a catalytic agent, an enzyme (so to speak), that will precipitate action.

In the report of the National Conference on Coordination of the School Health Program, titled *Teamwork in School Health*, the following patterns for coordination were proposed: "1. Informal procedures; 2. The ad-hoc problem-solving group; 3. The continuing committee or council; 4. The specialized advisory committee; 5. Combinations of adaptations of the foregoing." (1:7)

While each of the suggested patterns has merit and there will undoubtedly be occasion to use each of them, the continuing committee and council deserve special attention. The composition of each of the committees/councils and their working relationship is depicted in Figure 3. As indicated by the dotted line connecting the different levels, the relationship between the levels is a working relationship, not one of authority

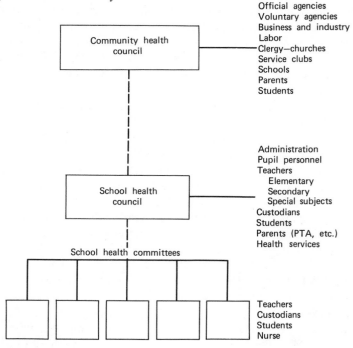

Figure 3. Community Organization for Coordination of the Health Education Program.

Without going into detail concerning the structure and function of the health councils and committees, we propose three levels of community action. These are not new, but they need implementation. The first, and universally possible, is the *school health committee*. As Dr. Cyrus Maxwell (8) pointed out several years ago, even in a one-teacher rural school there is need for such a committee. In such cases the school health committee may include the teacher, a pupil, a parent, a board member or trustee, a physician (possibly the health office), and a nurse (possibly a Public Health Nurse). It would be an action group, concerned with getting things done in and for a particular school or school building.

The second level of community action is the *school health council*. This council would be composed of school representatives in a given school system including representation from the school health committee. It would be concerned with philosophy and policies of the school system, not with carrying out any particular program. If a program is needed, it would be referred to the school health committee. The council would be strictly an advisory group, not an action group. The school health council is not intended to be representative of the entire community, just of the schools in the system. The school system might be a district, a township, a city, a county, or even a state.

The keystone of our bridge is the *community health council*. As is well known, the community health council will include representatives from many citizens' groups having a health interest. This will include representatives from the school health council, other school personnel, professional groups, civic groups, medical societies, voluntary health associations, governmental agencies, and many others. Like the school health council, the community health council is strictly an advisory body.

If, then, the various committees and councils form the building materials for our bridge, who serves as the engineer or supervisor to get the bridge constructed and who serves as the guide, gatekeeper, or catalyst, after it is built?

For these jobs we encourage the use of the *health coordinator*. It is well known that this term came into some disrepute at one time, and the term consultant was substituted. When that happened we began talking about another kind of job. We quit thinking of one dedicated to getting people to work together and began thinking, in many cases at least, of someone ready, willing, and able to give advice, supply information, and act as a resource person, but one who felt impelled to wait for a request for help. There is need for both consultant and coordinator, but at different levels of operation. The coordinator should be a local community level worker (Chapter 4) while the consultant may more logically work at the state level.

Some examples of the use of a health coordinator include the Kellogg program of the 1940s, the Los Angeles School System that employed nurses as coordinators in the 1950s, the Florida plan that required each school to designate a health coordinator in the late 1950s, and the Indiana law that made provision for employing qualified health coordinators by one or more school jurisdictions.

One of the first publications to refer to coordination of the school health program was *The Journal of School Health*. Palmeri (9) reported on a "School

64

District Health Council'' while Krigin and Glass (7) reported on ''A Student Health and Safety Council at Clayton Valley School.''

This same journal carried an article by Claude Cook (4), that supported the need for a health coordinator. The basis for this interpretation, in this light, is the conclusion that the health education teacher was perceived by the teacher, the principal, and the supervisor as a classroom instructor confined to the classroom. This is, of course, in direct contrast with the role of the health educator as envisioned by groups meeting in regional and national conferences and in conflict with a generally accepted principle of health education, that of extending the school or classroom activities into the community.

If this is a common perception of the work of the health educator, then someone must be designated to promote coordination. The health educator will not ordinarily be able to take the time from teaching nor will she/he be accepted unless specifically designated, or assigned, this responsibility. In some instances the supervisor may be performing this function, but too commonly the supervisor's interest and activity are limited to classroom instruction whereas the health coordinator must be concerned with all aspects of the school health program.

In addition to the use of committees, councils, and coordinating personnel, there should be more interchange between schools of public health and school health. More school health educators, specifically college and university health educators, should spend some time in a school of public health; and all school health personnel should have basic instruction in public health. Because many of them have been teachers, the public health education people may be fairly well informed on the nature and problems of school health; but as time goes on and as we get more public health educators without school teaching experience, this may not be the case. In fact, perhaps some of our present public health educators actually had an unpleasant school experience. If so, then a new look might do them good.

There should be more sharing of experiences at the professional preparation level, especially at the inservice level. Regular attendance at the conventions of The American School Health Association, the American Public Health Association, and the AAHPER should be encouraged and supported by the schools. However, this suggests another obstacle. How can the school health educator take the time and money to attend such a meeting? Schools do not generally provide released time and expense allowances for nonschool functions of this kind. The answer lies, in part at least, in the extent to which those present at national meetings carry back the message to others. This places a special responsibility on those who are in teacher education. It is for just such a purpose that the health educations graduate program in many institutions has courses dealing rather specifically with public health. Just as the good public health worker must be cognizant of the many facets of the community, including the school, the good school health worker must be aware of the many facets of the community outside the walls of the school. The typical public school classroom provides an excellent setting for bridging the gap. In this connection, *The Journal of School Health* is a valuable resource.

In proposing that a qualified health coordinator is best suited for the task of getting the gap bridged, we are not ignoring or belittling efforts of those who find it desirable to enlist the services of interested personnel who may lack some of the desirable qualifications. However, the philosophy that anything is better than nothing is questionable. In the case of the health coordinator, someone inadequately prepared might actually do more damage than good. There is need for school health and public health authorities to work together to establish minimum qualifications for the health coordinator and to work to secure the employment of such personnel.

Without attempting to list the special qualifications of the Coordinator, we can assume that he/she must understand both the school health and the public health programs. As indicated earlier, these two programs have much more in common than is usually recognized. The school health program is, in reality, an important aspect of the public health program. Although it differs from the program of the public health department, it is part of the concept of public health. We have done a grave disservice to the total public health program by creating this dichotomy, and it is time that we emphasize the unity.

Summary

With the various phases of the total school-community health program making their own individual unique contributions, we can look forward to greater achievements. Through the efforts of teachers who understand the public health program, in its broadest sense, we can develop a citizenry capable of participating in such a program. Under the leadership and stimulation of qualified health coordinators and other community leaders we can look forward to greater coordination and articulation of the several aspects of the public health program. Through the various systems of councils and committees that may be developed to meet community needs, we can secure a closer working relationship between all agencies so that we may more fully realize Winslow's concept of "preventing disease, prolonging life, and promoting health and efficiency through organized community effort." (3:3-4)

References

1. American Association for Health, Physical Education, and Recreation, *Teamwork in School Health*, AAHPER, Washington, D.C., 1962.

2. Castile, A.S. and S.J. Jerrick, "School Health in America: A Summary Report of State School Health Programs," *The Journal of School Health*, 46: 4 (1976).

3. Committee on Professional Education, "Educational Qualifications of Community Health Educators," *American Journal of Public Health*, 38: 6 (1948).

4. Cook, C.T., "Perceptions of the Functions and Competencies of Secondary School Health Educators," *The Journal of School Health,* 29: 2 (1959).

5. Hanlon, J.J., *Principles of Public Health Administration*, Mosby, St. Louis, 1974.

6. Ludwig, D.J. and J.K. Rash, "Preparation in Health Education Recommended for Majors in Physical Education." Presented at the Annual Meeting of the American Association for Health, Physical Education and Recreation, New York City, 1954.

7. Krigin, J. and L. Glass, "A Student Health and Safety Council at Clayton Valley School," *The Journal of School Health*, 29: 2 (1959).

8. Maxwell, C., "The Optimum School Health Program," *The Journal of School Health*, 20: 7 (1950).

9. Palmeri, J.F. "The School District Health Council: Is Its Existence Justified?" *The Journal of School Health*, 29: 2 (1959).

10. Ross, H.S., "Guidelines for the Preparation and Practice of Health Educators," *Health Education Monographs*, Society for Public Health Education, *5* (1) Spring 1977, pp. 75-81.

PART TWO
HEALTH EDUCATION CURRICULUM DESIGN

Chapter Seven
Principles of Curriculum Development in Health Education

Since the first attempts at formal education, curriculum planning and developing have been a responsibility of the people involved in the educative process. Choices of what to teach have always had to be made, and as the complexity of the educative process has increased so has the complexity of the curriculum development process. This is reflected in a Special Issue of *The Journal of School Health*. (14)

The American ideal of universal education has added immeasurably to the complexity of curriculum planning. This ideal, coupled with the ideal of a democratic society, has brought almost everyone related to either the school or the home into the process. It follows, then, that curriculum planners must make provision for including a wide range of individuals in curriculum development. It also follows that regardless of the contribution that can be made by state and/or federal agencies, the planning of a successful curriculum should remain a local responsibility.

The literature is replete with exhortations to involve wide community representation, as well as all disciplines within the school, in the curriculum development process.

Beauchamp suggested that there are three primary curriculum functions: curriculum *planning*, curriculum *implementation*, and curriculum *evaluation*. (2:204) Any successful curriculum development project must be concerned with all three functions. There must be planning at all levels of the curriculum; the planning will be concerned with (1) the total school curriculum, (2) the curriculum in the various divisions or disciplines such as health education; and (3) the development of special phases of the curriculum within a division, including the course of study and other plans to make the school health program educational.

In health education, the second level, planners will be concerned with all of the components of the health education curriculum. These components are the experiences in healthful living or the healthful environment, health services, health instruction in related courses, and the health education course(s) represented by the health education course of study.

One of the pioneers in curriculum planning, Franklin Bobbitt, suggested that

the first step of the educational engineer is to take a broad over-view of the entire field of man's life by way of seeing the major factors in perspective and in relation. On the basis of this preliminary over-view, he will plan the general route to be followed. This general route must be laid out before he is ready to undertake the accurate survey of the details. (3:2)

Since a broad overview is likely to raise more questions than it answers and since action cannot be taken on the basis of questions, it follows, as Bobbitt (3:3) indicated, that the tentative solutions to the questions raised must be the basis for curriculum development. Such solutions should be based on the best evidence available, and they should be subject to revision. Furthermore, the curriculum developers should not accept the judgement of others but should do their own evaluating and deciding.

The second step in curriculum construction is the identification of exact goals within the fields given in the overview and the specification of exact details of the procedure to be employed in reaching these goals. (3:4–5) While some goals have been identified (for example, the ability to read and write), there is still considerable uncertainty concerning many goals, especially in health education.

Much progress has been made in both of the above undertakings, but in our rapidly changing environment and culture there is no assurance that the goals identified in the past have remained, or should remain, as the goals for the present. It follows, then, that a continuous three step process of general overview, specific goal identification, and revision of goals be continued.

The three step process is particularly important in the new and rapidly changing field of health education. Not only do we live in a rapidly changing environment and culture, we are also dealing with a discipline in which the basic knowledge is being expanded at a phenomenally rapid pace. The discovery of antibiotics, marvelous though it was, really just opened the door in the field of health knowledge. The potential for intelligent self-direction of health behavior is constantly being expanded. To keep abreast of the new knowledge and to use it effectively, curriculum developers as well as all others concerned with health education must constantly evaluate and possibly modify their goals in the light of the new knowledge available to them.

General Principles of Curriculum Development

Since health education curriculum development is not unlike curriculum development in other disciplines, the following general principles will be helpful in the health education curriculum development program.

1. Education involves preparation for adult life.

The first general principle of curriculum development is that education is primarily preparation for adult life. Bobbitt suggested that

education is to prepare men and women for the activities of every kind which make up, or ought to make up, well-rounded adult life; that it has no other purpose; that everything should be done with a view to this purpose; and that nothing should be included which does not serve this purpose. (3:7–8)

In order for education to fulfill this purpose Bobbitt stated that

the first task is to discover the activities which ought to make up the lives of men and women; and along with these, the abilities and personal qualities necessary for proper performance. These are the educational objectives. (3:8)

While a number of present day educators would find fault with Bobbitt's emphasis on preparation for adult life, experience seems to confirm the need for an appropriate emphasis on the skills that are necessary for functioning in the adult world. Prominent among those essential skills are reading, simple arithmetic, oral and written expression, and elements of the scientific approach to problem solving. It is imperative that the needs and interests of children be considered and, for the most part, while meeting those needs and interests, the foundation is being laid for serving the adult. Thus, there is really no conflict between preparation for adult life and meeting the needs and interest of children. Furthermore, considerations such as community needs, legal requirements, and community mores must be taken into account.

The emphasis on behavioral objectives tends to favor focusing on the immediate needs of the student. However, the emphasis on strictly behavioral objectives is not universally accepted. Kneller advocated *specified* rather than behavioral objectives. (11:227) This may have special application in health education, since some of the expected outcomes may not be strictly behavioral. As Kneller pointed out, "certain specific content (or skills) could be required of all students at certain levels, and the students could be tested on how well they had acquired it." (loc cit) This might well apply to certain knowledge and practice outcomes. In the realm of attitudes, which are more difficult and sometimes undesirable to standardize, certain outcomes might be specified "in accordance with (a) a theory of knowledge and value adopted by the teacher himself, and (b) the talents and choices of the student." (loc cit) Kneller contended that adhering strictly to behavioral objectives tends to drastically circumscribe teaching and learning. Such an approach would not preclude the use of behavioral objectives, but it leaves room for both knowledge and attitudes objectives, both of which are basic to optimum health education. It is worthy of note that in referring to proper performance Bobbitt identified the need for the *competency* based instruction (Chapter 3) that is currently receiving considerable attention.

Bobbitt (3:8–10) suggested that through activity analysis, the broad range of human experiences should first be classified into major fields including *health activities*. Second, these experiences should be analyzed and categorized into more specific activities. Initially the activities should be divided into rather large units until the specific activities to be performed are identified. The specific activities will constitute the specific objectives of education.

While much of the work of classifying the specific activities has been accomplished and many desirable specific activities have been identified, the nature of health education dictates that curriculum planners continue to examine the activities in the light of the suggested criteria for selecting the desired expected outcomes (Chapter 13).

2. The success of a curriculum development project is related to the number and variety of people involved in the project.

Participation is the second principle fundamental to curriculum development. Simply stated, in order for curriculum development to make the optimum contribution to the school program, the greatest possible number of individuals must be involved. The experience of participating in the curriculum development process is as important as the resulting product, the curriculum guide.

The suggestion that as many people as possible should be involved in the curriculum development process was supported by Wiles (16), Tyler (15), and others. For example, Hass has said that

in America, all interested citizens, parents, learners and scholars from all of the disciplines must work with teachers, principals and supervisors in the planning. This planning should go on throughout America on a local, state and national basis. A democratic society cannot permit uniformity and centralization. (9:249)

It is especially important that those who may use the finished product, particularly the course of study, participate in the development process. A well- planned inservice education program regarding the use of the finished product can do much to counter the lack of participation for those not involved in the curriculum development process. Also, it is vital to the success of the curriculum project that both students and parents have an important part in developing the curriculum. To a great extent, the students and parents determine the success of the educational effort. It follows, then, that wide participation by students, parents, and teachers is essential.

Extensive discussion and related community education will be necessary to develop community understanding, agreement, and support for a comprehensive program of education. Health education is often very personal and sometimes it involves subject matter of a potentially controversial nature. Consequently, it is imperative that there be a free exchange of ideas and information among the members of the community: parents, teachers, students, and community leaders. Likewise, there should be a continuous process of community education to secure acceptance and approval of the kind of education that is essential for intelligent self-direction of health behavior in all aspects of life. Needless to say, not all members of the community will approve of education regarding certain aspects of life that may seem essential to others. Therefore, it is important to agree on what shall be taught in the controversial areas such as sex education, drugs, and socialized medicine. Through wide discussion and education it will be possible to arrive at decisions more widely acceptable than might otherwise be possible.

Goodlad indicated that

curriculum dialogue takes as its subject matter the ends and means of education and schooling: what shall be the over-all aims of education? What objectives shall the schools take for themselves? What is worth knowing? How shall the curriculum be organized? (8:91)

It follows that such questions will serve as the focus of wide community discussion and education.

Sound educational practice dictates that full consideration be given to important criteria for selecting what to include in the curriculum. The criteria of needs, interests, comprehension ability, possibility of independent action, and community values should be considered in planning for education that will lead to intelligent self-direction of student and adult health behavior.

As a result of wide discussion and community education, and in light of the preceding criteria, Bobbitt suggested that it will be possible to agree on which abilities (objectives) should be developed under the systematic care of the home, the church, and various other community agencies. Likewise, it can be determined which objectives should be left to the general process of living and which should be made the responsibility of the schools. (3:39)

3. The curriculum consists only of planned educational experiences.

Since students are constantly being subjected to many influences and are having a wide variety of experiences, it is important to realize just what comprises the curriculum. A third principle of curriculum development is *systematic planning*. It is important to note that the curriculum consists of the *planned* educative experiences and not everything that happens to a student. There are two common perceptions of curriculum that are in conflict with this principle. One is that the curriculum is confined to what happens in the classroom. The other is that all of the student's educational experiences make up the curriculum. Some of the many different experiences that may contribute to the education of students are not planned such as a serious accident, a preventable illness or a death. The curriculum should include plans for utilizing unplanned experiences in the total education process. Since many of them are not encouraged to happen, they are not dealt with in the curriculum.

Such systematically planned experiences need not always be under the direct supervision of the school but, if such experiences are to comprise a part of the curriculum there must be systematic planning for those experiences. It follows that if the results of such planning are to be available to teachers they must be in a form readily available to them over a period of time. This suggests that the curriculum should be in written form. This concept is supported by Hass who said ". . .the curriculum is a planned program based in part on prepared curriculum materials and planning by teachers and other professional staff members." (9:5)

4. The curriculum must reflect the value system of the community.

Smith, Stanley, and Shores stated that *few things are as important in curriculum development—and, indeed, in society generally—as a body of universal values on the basis of which important decisions can be made with the confidence that they will be favorably received. (13:59)*

They further indicated that "the values of people are the rules of conduct by which they shape their behavior and from which they derive their hopes. " (13:60) These comments suggest a fourth principle of curriculum development. *The curriculum must be developed in harmony with the value system of the community.* At the same time, however, the curriculum can and does exert a significant influence on that value system. This influence is brought to bear on the existing value system through the extensive community discussion and education previously mentioned; it cannot be imposed from without. Curriculum development that runs counter to the value system of the community is doomed to failure.

The current emphasis on *values clarification* and *behavior modification* results, in part, from the many failures experienced by people who have attempted to impose conflicting values through the curriculum development process. The imminent danger of attempts at values clarification rests in the temptation again to impose outside values, either on individuals or a community. It is claimed, with some degree of accuracy, that individuals must and do develop their own set of values. However, it must be recognized that no one develops a set of values completely independent of the environment, particularly in early childhood.

Christenson (4) reported that 84 percent of parents with children in public schools favored instruction that would deal with morals and moral behavior. The report clearly substantiates the view held by many curriculum scholars that the value system of a community is an important consideration in developing a curriculum and that it serves to give direction to such development.

The popularity of the *values clarification* movement may well be a manifestation of the desire for moral instruction, but Christenson indicated that it falls short of the kind of instruction needed. He stated:

High school students can be directly assisted in thinking more clearly about moral issues (as some teachers attempt to do), but teen-age attempts at value clarification are a wholly inadequate substitute for courses that forthrightly and lucidly explain what human experience over the centuries has taught us about some of the moral principles and attitudes that can enrich and profitably govern our lives. (4:739)

Christenson recommended a modernized revival of the McGuffey Reader Concept.

The criterion of *community values* must be considered in any curriculum development project, whether it be a simple course outline for a class or a complete revision of the total curriculum. Needless to say a set of universal values will be hard to develop, but the difficulty does not negate the need to make an attempt and to identify the best value system that can be achieved at the time.

Smith, Stanley, and Shores suggested that the core of the American system of values consists primarily of "The Democratic Tradition" (13:76) and "Maximum Development of the Individual" (13:79) and that

the core of the American system of values underlies most of the basic institutions of the nation. It is the ultimate justification of the public school system. . . .[T]he single-ladder system of universal education is based upon the doctrine of the supreme worth of the individual as an object of development. (13:81)

These authors further suggested that

[T]he fundamental principles comprising the core of American culture must become objects of study in the same sense and to the same degree that the principles of science are now studied. (13:83)

77

5. Progress in education is made slowly.

The current emphasis on values clarification appears to be one belated move in a direction suggested some 20 years earlier. This move illustrates the principle that *progress in the educational system comes about slowly*. It is recognized that a period of approximately 30 years ordinarily elapses between the time when an innovation in education is generally recognized as being desirable and when it is considered to have somewhat universal application. In light of this experience, it must be recognized that large scale curriculum reform will come about slowly, but individual schools and school systems need not be discouraged from undertaking innovations in their curriculum development. On the contrary, significant curriculum reform can only be made in this manner. However, it would be a mistake to assume that large scale acceptance of such innovations would follow immediately. This principle has further implications in health education that will be discussed later.

In summary, at least five general principles should serve to guide curriculum development. Briefly stated they are: (1) education is primarily preparation for adult life; (2) the success of a curriculum development project is directly related to the number and variety of people involved; (3) the curriculum consists *only* of planned educative experiences; (4) the curriculum must be developed in harmony with the value system of the community; and (5) progress in the education system takes place slowly.

Using these five general principles as guidelines, curriculum developers should next look for specific principles that may serve as guidelines in their respective areas of education.

Principles with Special Application to Health Education

In developing the health education curriculum, it is important to consider each of the general principles outlined above. In addition, it is important to consider specific principles with direct application to health education. These principles might be thought of as *principles of health education*, and as such they serve as guiding rules in the development of the health education curriculum.

1. Learning is an inherent drive.

The first principle of health education to consider is that *learning is an inborn, inherent drive of the human organism*. Children are born to learn: knowledge, attitudes, and practices (habits and skills). Given a normally healthful climate, they grow in physical stature, emotional maturity, the use of social skills, and spiritual well-being. Developmental tasks, as suggested by Cushman (5), also

78

motivate learning: for example, adjusting to a new baby in the family, adjusting. to school, adjusting to college life, and other tasks.

As Allport (1) suggested, growth is enhanced through the setting of long range goals that are value oriented. This concept is especially true for emotional and spiritual growth. The importance of goals is supported by the Toronto study (1968–1970) (12) in which it was discovered that normlessness, the absence of norms or goals, was directly related to the incidence of drug use among the 15,312 youths studied.

Recognizing that learning is an inherent drive and that learning is enhanced by setting goals, curriculum developers can shape the curriculum to take advantage of these two important facts.

2. Positive example promotes the development of sound health practices.

The second principle of health education is that *children learn from example.* This principle is especially true of younger children. As Hochbaum pointed out, the family is the social unit that exerts the most direct and profound influence on the children. The intimate contacts and shared experiences mitigate in the direction of accepted attitudes and practices. As Hochbaum said, "These health attitudes are passed on by parents to their children, partly intentionally, partly through their examples, and partly in various subtle and imperceptible ways of which neither they nor the children are aware." (10:48)

The role of family influence in drug use was supported by Smart and Fejer (12:8) in their report on trends in drug use among adolescents. They reported a consistent relationship between the use of drugs by parents and their children. Hochbaum also pointed out that in cases where children deliberately go against parental standards and remain nonsmokers or become teetotalers, their behavior is "clearly as much due to their relationship with their parents as if they had followed their parents' examples." (10:49) Hence the exemplar role of parents, siblings, peers, teachers, and heroes is important in the lives of children.

Nelson Bradley, M.D.* medical director of the Lutheran General Hospital Rehabilitation Center at Park Ridge, Illinois, has suggested that the following traits, which he considers important in the therapist, are also the same traits important in the teacher. The effective therapist (or teacher) is a warm, loving, genuine person; empathetic; nonjudgmental; honest; charismatic; action oriented; and spiritually comfortable. These traits not only serve to make the teacher or therapist more effective, but they help the subject set personal goals through ex-

---

* Lecture at the Workshop on Problems of Alcoholism, Alcohol Education, and Drug Misuse, Indiana University, Bloomington, June 12, 1973.

ample. Example continues to be one of the most important factors in influencing behavior.

3. Early childhood learnings tend to persist.

The third principle of health education is that *patterns, (physical, emotional, social, and spiritual) are so well established by the time the child comes to school it is difficult to change them.* This principle is supported by Hochbaum (10) and by Galdston who cited the World Health Organization Monograph, *Maternal Care and Mental Health* which supported the thesis that "any young child denied the presence, the care, and the affection of its mother is by that deprivation deleteriously affected from the remainder of its life." (7:11)

The school enters the development scene so late in the life of the child that remedial education becomes its principal task. Thus the school must foster unlearning as part of the learning process. A long range goal of health education should be the establishment of desirable health practices in infancy and early childhood. Since this goal can only be accomplished by the parents, it becomes necessary for the schools to focus on preparation for parenthood and to include programs of education of parents and prospective parents. Throughout all phases of education it must be recognized that health practices are well established in early life.

4. Thorndykes' principles of learning: readiness, exercise, and effect apply in health education.

The fourth principle of health education is that *readiness, exercise, and effect are important considerations in health instruction.* In recent years there have been several attempts to update or modernize the principles (laws) of learning suggested by Thorndyke. For the most part such attempts have resulted in little more than new terminology applied to well-established principles.

In simple terms the principle of *readiness* recognizes that there is a psychologically opportune time for a particular learning: when the individual feels a need to know or do. The principle of *exercise* recognizes that learnings are strengthened through exercise or repetition. It should be emphasized that undesirable learnings are acquired in the same manner as are desirable ones. We learn by doing! The principle of *effect* recognizes that the act tends to be repeated when and if the experience is pleasant, but not that pleasant experiences are remembered better.

The desirability of a practice from a health-related standpoint probably has little influence on consistent practice. If the goal of total unhealthful behavior were sought, it would probably be just as difficult to achieve as the goal of totally healthful behavior.

80

5. A favorable environment promotes learning.

The fifth principle of health education states *there can be an environment that is conducive to learning.* The role of the teacher is frequently discussed and sometimes maligned. It is commonly recognized that the teacher is the most important influence in the classroom, but there is less agreement concerning the specific functions of the teacher. Since there can be an environment that is conducive to learning, the proper function of teaching is to foster such an environment. This suggests the need to consider a different definition of teaching. Perhaps teaching should be defined as *fostering an environment that is conducive to learning.* Teachers cannot force learning on the individual because the individual must do the learning. The teacher must recognize this. Frazer has quoted Comenius as having said, over 3000 years ago, "To teach well is to enable someone to learn rapidly, agreeably, and thoroughly." (6:5)

In an analysis of the definition of teaching as fostering an environment that is conducive to learning, there are probably five specific considerations for the teacher: (1) to provide a favorable physical environment; (2) to foster a favorable emotional environment; (3) to inform, that is, to present new facts and ideas not otherwise available to the learners, (4) to inspire or motivate, and (5) to interpret or explain. If the capable teacher focuses on these functions the result will very likely be an environment that encourages learning.

6. Reinforcement is conducive to positive learning.

The sixth principle of health education is that *learning may be enhanced by reinforcement.* Positive reinforcement is usually most effective, but there are times for negative reinforcement. Such negative reinforcement need not be in the form of punishment. It may, in fact, be the simple removal of a support, such as keeping forbidden objects out of sight of young children.

About 100 years ago a newsletter of the (Indiana) State Charities Aid Association contained the suggestion that every vice is a perverted virtue; if the virtue is cultivated, the vice no longer prevails. This concept suggests the desirability of reinforcing the desirable behavior of the young child while largely ignoring (negatively reinforcing) undesirable behavior.

7. The perception of the individual influences learning.

The seventh principle of health education is that *people react to their perception* of what they hear or see and not to what is said or done. Two people will almost invariably perceive the same event differently. What might be perceived favorably by one person might well be perceived by another as a threat. Percep-

81

tion may depend on the interpretation or understanding of words, or it may arise from cultural differences; for example, in some cultures milk is not considered potable because the cow is sacred, whereas the use of powdered milk might be acceptable. Since perception is the key factor, it becomes imperative that perceptions be clarified. Likewise, it is especially important that teachers determine how the learner perceives an experience.

8. Health learning may not be immediately applicable and may not result in an immediate change in behavior.

The eighth principle of health education is that *there may be considerable delay between learning and application.* The practical application of much of the learning in health education is, of necessity, not possible for some time after the initial learning takes place. This fact is especially true of the learning related to the recognition of disease, to long-time effects of diet and of stress, and to the health needs related to child bearing and child rearing.

For example, young adults may learn the danger signals of cancer, but in all probability it will be 20 to 30 years before they will have the actual need to be able to recall and recognize those signs. Similarly, in health or home economics classes in high school students may have learned about child care but, except for babysitters and those who help care for siblings, few will apply that learning until they have their own family some years in the future.

While many cannot accept the thesis that it is not necessary to learn facts that can be readily researched, knowing where to find such facts is often as important as knowing the facts. Similarly, the knowledge underlying principles of health conservation is more important than the simple health facts.

Summary

There are at least eight principles that have special application to health education and to health education curriculum development. These are: (1) the principle that learning is an inherent drive, (2) exemplar principle, (3) primacy principle, (4) Thorndyke's principles of learning: readiness, exercise, and effect, (5) favorable environment principle, (6) reinforcement principle, (7) perception principle, and (8) delayed response principle.

Consideration of each of these principles will help to ensure the development of a more effective curriculum in health education.

References

1. Allport, G.W., *Becoming*, Yale University, New Haven, 1955.

2. Beauchamp, G.A., *Curriculum Theory*, Third Edition, Kagg, Willmette, Illinois, 1975.

3. Bobbitt, Franklin, *How to Make A Curriculum*, Houghton, Chicago, 1924.

4. Christenson, R.M., "McGuffey's Ghost and Moral Education Today," *Phi Delta Kappan*, 58:10 (1977).

5. Cushman, W.P., "Developmental Tasks—A Source of Health Problems," *The Journal of School Health*, 29:7 (1959).

6. Frazer, Alexander, Editor, *A Curriculum for Children*, Association for Supervision and Curriculum Development, Washington, D.C., 1969.

7. Galdston, Iago, M.D., *Beyond the Germ Theory*, Health Education Council, New York and Minneapolis, 1954.

8. Goodlad, J.I., R. von Steophasius, and M.F. Klein, *The Changing School Curriculum*, The Fund for the Advancement of Education, New York, 1966.

9. Hass, Glen, "Who Should Plan the Curriculum?" in Glen Hass, J. Bondi, and J. Wiles, *Curriculum Planning, A New Approach*, Allyn, Boston, 1970.

10. Hochbaum, G.M., *Health Behavior*, Wadsworth, 1970.

11. Kneller, G.F., "Behavioral Objectives? No!" in Hass, G., J. Bondi, and J. Wiles, *Curriculum Planning, A New Approach*, Allyn, Boston, 1970.

12. Smart, R.G. and D. Fejer, *Recent Trends in Drug Use Among Adolescents*, Canada's Mental Health Supplement, May–August, 1971.

13. Smith, B.O., W.O. Stanley, and J.H., Shores, *Fundamentals of Curriculum Development*, World, New York, 1957.

14. "Special Issue: Design and Implementation of School Health Curricula," *The Journal of School Health* 48:4 (1978).

15. Tyler, R.W., *Basic Principles of Curriculum and Instruction*, University of Chicago, Chicago, 1974, c1949.

16. Wiles, K., "Seeking Balance in the Curriculum," in Hass, G., J. Bondi, and J. Wiles, *Curriculum Planning, A New Approach*, Allyn, Boston, 1970.

Chapter Eight
Organization for Health Education Curriculum Development

In discussing the organization needed to develop or plan the health education curriculum we are concerned with what is commonly called curriculum engineering, which involves the essential processes of a curriculum system. The three primary functions of curriculum engineering are "(1) to produce a curriculum, (2) to implement the curriculum, and (3) to appraise the effectiveness of the curriculum and the curriculum system." (2:135) These are the functions essential to the success of a curriculum development process.

The responsibility for planning and implementing the development of the curriculum rests largely with the curriculum engineers, but this does not minimize the importance of teacher initiative and teacher involvement. The initiative for developing or revising the curriculum might logically come from the teachers. As indicated earlier, teachers, parents, and students should make up the nucleus of the curriculum development team, but it should also include representatives of interested community groups. If many people are to be involved, there must be a plan of organization that will allow for the most effective participation of each person. It is this organization of personnel with which we are now concerned.

In planning the health education curriculum designed *to provide the systematic organization of courses, and other activities, experiences, and situations,* as specified in our accepted definition, we must call on all available community resources. This is imperative to ensure that all points of view be brought into the curriculum and that the full cooperation of all concerned be enlisted for the development and functioning of the curriculum. The importance of such participation by administrators, supervisors, teachers, parents, and students is supported by such curriculum scholars as Beauchamp (2:176, 1:285–301), Tyler (4:126), Smith, Stanley, and Shores (3:451–452), and others. Although the process of

85

developing a curriculum will take longer when there is wide community participation, it is also agreed that a good curriculum development project must be carried on slowly and deliberately.

It is a well-established principle of learning that identification with an idea, or ideal, comes from, or is coeval with, participation in the development of that idea or ideal. The full cooperation of a community can only be enjoyed when the community feels that it has had a part in planning and developing the program in which the cooperation is desired. As a corollary to securing the cooperation of the community, the educational value to those who participate in the planning is an important outcome of the process.

When the cooperation of a community is enjoyed, that cooperation may be expressed in many ways such as interest in and encouragement of new ideas and new methods of teaching, defense of school personnel against unjust criticism, giving constructive criticism based on careful examination of the facts, and through joint effort in carrying out the program.

The development of the health education curriculum through joint planning procedures will, of necessity, be slower than if planned by so-called experts. Furthermore, it is important to be realistic and to recognize that it is more difficult to please many than a few. The result is that some aspects of the curriculum may not seem important or appropriate to the group doing the planning. Consequently, the results may not include everything that seems important to each individual. Planning does not stop with agreement on a tentative curriculum. It is a continuous process. The omission of what may seem like important points at first should stimulate further discussion and education. This should lead to further consideration of controversial points as the curriculum is used, evaluated, and revised.

Since the health education curriculum includes the educational experiences afforded through health services, the healthful environment, and other courses, provision must be made for ensuring that students have those experiences. It is also important that the representatives of these services be involved in planning the curriculum.

The nature and content of the health education curriculum manual might follow this outline:

Health Education Curriculum Manual

1. The philosophy of the school regarding health education, its role in education, and administrative and legal provisions for the program.
2. The definition of curriculum that is accepted.
3. The components of the health education curriculum: health services, healthful environment, related courses, and health education courses.

4. The broad educational outcomes desired, including a statement of long range goals as they relate to the needs and interests of both the students and the members of the community.

5. Detailed plans (the instructional guides) for each of the four aspects of the health education curriculum.

   A. Role of health services, including a statement of philosophy regarding the role of health services, educational outcomes, and evaluation procedures.

   B. Role of healthful environment, including philosophy, services, educational outcomes, and evaluation procedures.

   C. Role of related courses, including philosophy, designated courses, educational outcomes, and evaluation procedures.

   D. Role of the health education courses, the health education course of study.

6. Provision for evaluating and revising the curriculum.

Basic Considerations In Curriculum Planning

Joint planning for the health education curriculum involves 10 basic considerations. These are:

1. Administrative support
2. The curriculum project coordinator
3. The health education curriculum advisory council
4. The health education curriculum committee
5. The central course of study committee
6. The instructional unit committees
7. The tryout personnel and procedure
8. Editing and publishing the course of study
9. Distribution of the course of study
10. Evaluation and revision of the course of study

administrative support

The success of the health education curriculum in achieving the goals of health education depends to a very great extent on the willingness and ability of the administration to provide moral and material support. Such willingness does not guarantee success because the program must be planned and carried out by will-

87

ing, intelligent, and well-prepared personnel. However, the absence of such support makes the work of the personnel much more difficult and the results much slower. If there is absence of the support of the administration the first step in curriculum development would, of necessity, be the systematic and deliberate attempt to win the interest and support essential to success. In the meantime individual teachers are at all times obligated to review and improve that aspect of the curriculum with which they are concerned, their own individual efforts.

the curriculum project coordinator

With the support of the administration as the representative of the school board, the selection of a health education curriculum project coordinator would be an early step. Since the administration must at all times be close to the project and must be kept informed of the progress, a representative of administration might be the logical choice for the project coordinator. Individuals in the following positions would be logical candidates for this position: assistant superintendent, curriculum director, or a principal. The absence of the health coordinator, director, or supervisor from this list is deliberate, since the efforts of this person can be most effective working back stage, on a person-to-person basis, stimulating thought and activity, ironing out problems, securing and distributing new materials, etc. In other words, by working behind the scenes to ensure the continuity and effectiveness of the project.

The chief criteria for the selection of the project coordinator are interest in the growth and development of the total school program, knowledge of principles of curriculum development, and ability to participate in a project that is being developed through the group process.

The project coordinator will not be personally responsible for the creative planning dealing with technical health information. In view of the special abilities needed and of the time to be devoted to the project it is important that the person be a member of the school staff.

the health education curriculum advisory council

The health education curriculum advisory council is one of four important functional bodies concerned with the curriculum project. The others are the health education curriculum committee, the central course of study committee, and the instructional unit committee(s), one for each grade or major grade level for which unit plans are being constructed. The inter-relationship of these committees is shown in Figure 4.

Three important broad functions of the health education curriculum advisory council are: (1) to provide resources from which to draw in determining the health education needs and interests of pupils as well as the community health needs; (2) to provide opportunity for increasing the understanding and apprecia-

88

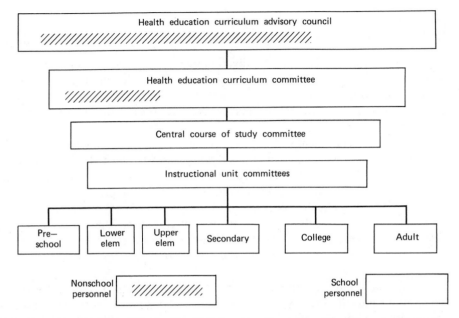

Figure 4. Organization Plan for Health Education Curriculum Development Project.

tion of the community as they relate to health and the school health program; and (3) to secure support for the conduct and growth of the program and for meeting unfair or unjustified criticism. If the council is to fulfill these functions, it must represent the entire school community.

The more specific responsibilities of the health education curriculum advisory council would fall in the major categories of development of philosophy and policy formulation. Specifically, it might be charged with responsibility for:

1. Developing statements of philosophy concerning the nature of the health program.

2. Determining the principal health and health education needs of the community.

3. Determining the principal health education needs of the pupils.

4. Deciding some areas of health education outcomes to be stressed in schools.

5. Determining general policies concerning development and application of the health education curriculum.

6. Acquainting the public with the needs and progress of the school health curriculum project.

7. Surveying the opportunities for coordination of efforts of all health workers.

8. Stimulating a keen interest in the project.

9. Acting as a consultant group for the health education curriculum committee.

The criteria for selection of individual members of the advisory council are: interest, backround (education or experience), official designation, health interest of parent organization. It is important that there be representation of all important local organizations and agencies having a concern for and interest in the health of the citizens.

The close relationship of the school health program and the community health program must be recognized, as discussed in Chapter 5. In this connection the role of the community health educator or coordinator becomes important. This person provides the vital communication link in the program. In cooperation with the school health coordinator (or department head) and representatives of other community health agencies, a study of community health resources and needs can be carried out. Parents can be involved in a study of student health needs and interests. In this manner the role of the advisory council can be enhanced.

The community health council or the health division or committee of the community council, might well serve as the advisory council for the health education curriculum development project. In such cases it would be advisable to have additional representatives from the school serving as temporary or ex-officio members of the council during such time as health education curriculum problems were receiving attention.

If there is not an active community council, a special health education curriculum advisory council should be developed. The selection of the most appropriate individuals to serve on the council is of vital importance. It should be the prerogative of each agency to select its own representatives. However, it is the responsibility of the school to provide such leadership and guidance, including information concerning the duties of the representatives, as is needed to secure satisfactory representation of each agency.

Membership on the advisory council should be representative of the following agencies and organizations:

Official Agencies
Health Department
Public Welfare
Fire Department
Police Department
Schools

Government
City
County

Voluntary Agencies
Cancer Society
Society for the Crippled
Heart Association
The National Foundation, Inc.
Red Cross
Lung Association
Mental Health Association
Social Health Association
Council on Family Relations

90

Professional Associations
Dental
Medical
Nursing
Ministerial

Labor and Management
Unions
Manufacturers association

Parent-Teacher-Student
Associations

Civic and Service Clubs
American Legion
Chamber of commerce
Women's club
Fraternities and Sororities
with health interest
Service clubs
Senior Citizens clubs

The officers of the Council would probably consist of president, vice-president, and secretary. There might be some significat advantage in enlisting support of the project among key groups if the president and vice-president were representative of the medical society and of the parents of the community. During the period of the curriculum development project it would be desirable to have a member of the school staff serve as secretary to provide the important link between the council, the curriculum committee, and the central course of study committee. Furthermore, the work of the secretary is so extensive as to place unusually heavy demands on the time of a volunteer.

health education curriculum committee

While the role of the advisory council is strictly advisory, there must be an official body charged with the responsibility of overseeing the development of the total curriculum, including the development of courses of study, plans for coordinating the instruction in other courses with the health education classes, use of the educational opportunities in the health services offered by the school, and use of the educational opportunities in the healthful living program (the healthful environment) of the school. The Health Education Curriculum Committee has the responsibility for supervising the development of all aspects of the health education curriculum.

This committee serves as the representative of the school board, through the administrators; hence it reports to the board, either directly or through the administrator, as the situation warrants.

The personnel of the health education curriculum committee will consist of representatives from all aspects of the school health program, a few key community representatives, selected teachers who are not directly concerned with health education, students, representatives of the administration, and representatives of the parent-teacher-student association. It is important that some members of this committee also be on the advisory council and some on the central course of study committee.

91

Membership on the health education curriculum committee should be representative of the following:

School Health Program
Health education teachers
Custodians
School nurse
School physicial
Nutritionist
Supervisor of health education
Health coordinator

Administration
Curriculum director
Elementary school principal
Secondary school principal

Nonhealth Teachers
Biology
Social studies
Physical education
Elementary school
Secondary school

P.T.S.A./O.
Chairman of health commission
Interested parents
Students

Community Representatives
Health department
Voluntary agencies
Medical society
Dental society

The only officers needed for this committee are a chairperson and a secretary. It would not be a wise procedure to select the curriculum director, the supervisor of health education, or the health coordinator to serve as an officer since these individuals should be active in promoting the development of the curriculum without being in a so-called official position as far as the project committee is concerned. Also, in the interest of efficiency, it might be desirable to use one of the professional secretaries, possibly one from the office of the curriculum director.

the central course of study committee

The central course of study committee is responsible for the ultimate development of the health education course of study. While teachers will do most of the actual work of developing the instructional units, it is the responsibility of this committee to supervise the process.

The health education course of study is *a guide prepared for use by teachers, supervisors, administrators, and others with responsibilities for health education.* It is systematically organized by units of instruction for the designated grades; with expected outcomes; content; methods, devices, and techniques; teaching aids or supplies and equipment; references; and procedures for evaluating the outcomes suggested for direct instruction for health.

The direct health instruction program, as ordinarily outlined in a course of study, comprises the heart of the school health education curriculum. The contributions of the other phases of the curriculum, health services, healthful school living, and health instruction in related areas, are all important in the health education of pupils. However, the course of study, as the official guide, occupies the key position in the health instruction efforts of the school.

Since the course of study is to be used by virtually all health education personnel there should be wide sharing of responsibilities for developing the guide. It would be unrealistic to expect many persons who are not employed by the school to devote the time necessary to serving on the central course of study committee. However, it is important that all phases of the curriculum be represented in the development of the course of study.

The chief responsibilities of the central course of study committee are:

1. To provide the general pattern for the development of the various units of the course of study.

2. To select major problem areas and broad concepts to be included in the course of study.

3. To determine the course of study project calendar. This is normally a three year project, under favorable conditions, allowing one year for development, one year for tryout of instruction units, and one year for revision, editing, publishing, and distribution.

4. To estimate the time budget of each working member and recommend adjustment of work load accordingly.

5. To serve as a clearinghouse to avoid duplication, prevent omission of important problem areas, and to assist in resolving differences and conflicts between committees or between committee members.

6. To be responsible for arranging for tryout of the units and for final editing, publication, and distribution of the course of study.

7. To provide the organization necessary to ensure constant study, evaluation, and periodic revision of the course of study.

The personnel of the central course of study committee should include the chairman of each of the instructional unit committees. The officers of the committee should include a chairman, vice-chairman, and secretary. It is important that some of the school personnel on the health education curriculum committee also be on the central course of study committee, thus allowing for better articulation between the two committees.

Membership on the central course of study committee should be representative of the following positions or services of the school:

Nonteaching personnel: Health services, students, parents, custodian, lunch program manager, and student counselor.

93

Administrative staff: Superintendent or assistant, secondary school principal, elementary school principal, health coordinator, and health education supervisor.

Types of teachers: Elementary grades, biology, general science, home economics, physical education, safety education, and health education.

Two principles that would function in selection of teachers to serve on this committee are: (1) The teacher should be particularly well suited to a course-of-study development as judged by the teacher's backround, experience, and ability to work cooperatively. (2) A wide variety of schools should be represented, preferably of diverse geographic, economic, and social backrounds.

There should be appropriate modification of the size of the central course of study committee for the extremely small or exceptionally large school systems. In the small school system there might be more than one representative from a school, while in the exceptionally large city it would not be possible to have all schools or all types of teachers represented on the committee.

the instructional unit committees

The responsibility for preparing the specific instructional or resource units rests with the instructional unit committee. This is the working committee. Development of instructional units may follow either of two patterns. The committees that develop the units may function according to *subject matter* or *grade level.* In the first pattern a committee would develop the desired units for an instructional area, such as family living, for all grade levels in which such instruction is to be offered. In the second pattern a committee would develop the desired units for a particular grade level, such as for the intermediate grades, including units for all instructional areas or broad concepts for which such instruction is to be offered at that grade level. Either of these approaches allows for a wide range of flexibility in selecting the unit areas, ranging from the traditional health problem areas to broad concepts or principles that may be developed.

The subject matter committee, as stated, would prepare units in only one subject matter area. It would prepare these units for each grade or major grade level in which such instruction was desired. The membership of such a committee would include subject matter specialists as well as persons with a good understanding of the special needs, interests, and comprehension abilities of children of different ages. Such a committee would facilitate the articulation of instruction from grade to grade, for the area. Such articulation would be particularly helpful in developing a course of study along the cycle plan.

The grade level committee would prepare units for only one major grade level. It would prepare units in each of the problem areas in which instruction was desired at that grade level. The membership of the grade level committee would include teachers of that particular grade or major grade level, teachers from adjacent grades, and subject matter specialists for each instructional area for which units are to be developed. Such a committee would facilitate the meeting of the needs, interests, and comprehension abilities of the children with whom they are best acquainted. Articulation from grade to grade would, in this instance, be worked out in meeting with the central course of study committee and/or the other instructional unit committees.

The course of study is ordinarily thought of as the guide for instruction in the health education classes. However, as our definition indicates, it is for use by anyone who has responsibility for health education. This includes members of the health service team and the environmental health staff. Thus it is important that plans be made for ensuring that the opporutnies for health education in these related areas be utilized. This will include plans similar to unit plans that give guidance to nurses, dentists, physicians, environmental engineers, custodians, matrons, locker room attendants, etc. Needless to say, a program of inservice education will be mandated. These plans should be worked out by committees that include representatives of the profession concerned, along with teachers who have rapport with the staff that is involved. The focus of these plans will be on the common day-to-day experiences of the students, such as the physical examinations, first aid, the school lunch, and safety on the playground.

Selection of the personnel to be part of the instructional or resource unit committees will ordinarily be made on the basis of the criteria of preparation, willingness, availability, and ability to work as a member of the group. A working committee of from five to nine members would be considered desirable. Resource materials and personnel should be available to the committee at all times. This committee will ordinarily be made up of teachers.

Since professional growth of the participants in the development of the course of study is a major objective, it is important that sufficient time be allowed for the project. The educational value to all concerned depends largely on allowing adequate time for the project. If possible, the members of the instructional or resource unit committees should be allowed released time for the work of preparing the unit plans. This might be accomplished through summer employment for the members of the committee. However, this would tend to keep the committee small because of the expense involved. If released time or reduction of teaching load cannot be provided to the members of these committees, this should be recognized by reduction of teaching load or of co-curricular responsibilities and modification of the time schedule for developing the course of study.

In unit development, it is particularly important that the plans be developed through group discussion. Various group processes may be utilized, but *brainstorming* is one of the most fruitful. The uninhibited listing of thoughts, later to be evaluated, often turns up ideas that prove to be extremely valuable. This has special application in identifying health problem areas and in methodology. If the members of the group participate actively and conscientiously, the product will be noticeably superior to that resulting from a compilation of individual ideas and efforts and, furthermore, the professional growth of each participant will be significantly greater. However, decision making through group discussion is a time-consuming procedure, a fact that must be taken into consideration in setting up the project schedule.

The functions of the council and of the committees may be summarized as follows:

The advisory council: Counseling

The curriculum committee: Planning and implementing

The course of study committee: Directing

The instructional unit committees: Constructing

It is worthy of special note that communication between levels (council and committees) is essential to the success of the curriculum project. To facilitate such communication each committee should have representation on the next superior body. For example, a representative of each instruction unit committee might well be a member of the central course of study committee, several persons from the central course of study committee might be on the health education curriculum committee, and some from that committee might be on the advisory council.

These functions, or responsibilities, are shown in Figure 5.

the tryout personnel and procedures

Since the course of study will be in some printed form and will be used for several years, although distinctly tentative, it should be refined as much as possible. After careful preparation by experienced and skilled teachers, the units should be subjected to tryouts by teachers of proven ability along with some beginning teachers. A program of inservice education should be provided for the tryout teachers to acquaint them with the units to be tested and to instruct them in the tryout procedures and subsequent reporting.

More preliminary units should be prepared than are needed for the course of study. These preliminary units should be tried out with typical classes by skilled teachers who are informed concerning the purpose of the tryout and who are acquainted with important points to be noted and reported. These points include pupil response; pupil growth; time needed for the unit; adequacy of estimates of supplies and equipment; suitability of evaluation procedures; appropriateness of expected outcomes and content; and general quality of the units.

Health Education Curriculum Advisory Council (Community Representatives)	
1. General philosophy	5. Aim
2. Policies	6. Broad expected outcomes
3. Needs	7. Resources
4. Purposes	8. Support

Health Education Curriculum Committee (School and Committee Representatives)	
1. Health education philosophy	5. Supervise
2. Plan	6. Evaluate
3. Promote	7. Revise
4. Coordinate	8. Adjudicate
	9. Publish curriculum

Central Course of Study Committee, (School Representatives)	
1. Health education philosophy	7. Scheduling
2. Broad expected outcomes	8. Approval
3. Procedures	9. Tryout
4. Responsibilities	10. Revision
5. Scope	11. Publication
6. Broad content areas	12. Evaluation

Unit Committees (Teachers)	
1. Philosophy	5. Methods, devices, and techniques
2. Problem areas	6. Teaching aids
3. Expected outcomes	7. Evaluation procedures
4. Content	8. References

Figure 5. Functional Chart for Health Education Curriculum Development Project.

It is highly desirable that several different teachers try each unit in situations that provide for typical unhurried use. Ordinarily the tryout period should extend over the full time for which the course of study is planned. Adequate time allows for teacher preparation, thorough presentation, exchange of experiences with other teachers, and a critical evaluation of the whole process.

Teachers who have tried out the units should meet with the committee that prepared the unit to report their experiences and to offer criticisms and suggestions for revisions. The committee, working with the tryout teachers, should then make desirable revisions or reject units that do not seem worthy of revision. When the final refined course of study is ready for publication, provision must then be made for editing, publishing, and distributing it and for subsequent evaluation and revision. This will be discussed in Chapter 11.

The evaluation and revision committee should include representatives of the teachers who are using the guide, the health education coordinator, or supervisor, and students. Committee members must be cognizant of new developments, both in education and in health.

Evaluation of the total school health education program will be discussed in Chapter 20. Evaluation of the course of study should follow some of the same procedures. However, the primary concerns in this instance focus on the adequacy of the guide in assisting teachers. There needs to be a planned system of reporting needed revisions by teachers and students who are using the guide. Specific individuals should be charged with the responsibility of reporting new developments. The committee should meet regularly to assess the situation and to make recommendations for implementing the necessary revisions whether it be sections of the guide or a complete revision. No more than five years should elapse before a complete revision is undertaken.

Summary

There are distinct advantages in the cooperative development of the health education curriculum involving both the school and community representatives. The health interests of the community should be considered in the overall planning while all aspects of the school should be represented. This includes the health services, the healthful environment, health education courses, and related courses, as well as the students and their parents.

If a large and diverse number of people are to be involved in developing the health education curriculum, an effective plan of organization and procedure is essential. The plan outlined in this chapter provides one basis for planning for such an undertaking.

References

1. Beauchamp, G. A., *The Curriculum of the Elementary School*, Allyn, Boston, 1964.
2. Beauchamp, G. A., *Curriculum Theory*, Kagg, Willmette, Illinois, 1975.

3. Smith, B. O., W. O. Stanley, and J. H. Shores, *Fundamentals of Curriculum Development*, Revised Edition, World, Yonkers-on-Hudson, 1975.
4. Tyler, R. W., *Basic Principles of Curriculum and Instruction*, The University of Chicago, Chicago, 1974, c1949.

Chapter Nine
The Fundamental Nature of the Health Education Curriculum

It is generally agreed that the school is the chief educational agency in the community and that teaching is the main responsibility of the school. Furthermore, teaching is too commonly perceived as imparting knowledge. However, the modern concept of teaching and learning goes far beyond the acquisition of knowledge. This is especially true in health education. For this reason we are suggesting a different definition of teaching. As we perceive it, *teaching is fostering an environment that is conducive to learning.* It is to this end that curriculum development in health education should be directed.

Beauchamp has indicated that the field of curriculum has two parts: curriculum design and curriculum engineering. (1:195) One aspect of curriculum engineering was discussed in Chapter 7. In the field of curriculum design we must be concerned with an understanding of the nature of curriculum if we are to approach intelligently the task of planning an effective curriculum.

Definitions of Curriculum

Several definitions of curriculum have been suggested. Smith et al. described curriculum as:

> *A set of potential experiences . . . set up in the school for the purpose of disciplining children and youth in group ways of thinking and acting. (4:3)*

They stated further that:

> *The curriculum is always, in every society, a reflection of what the people think, feel, and do. (4:3)*

In the *Dictionary of Education*, Good defined curriculum as:

A body of prescribed educative experiences under school supervision, designed to provide an individual with the best possible training and experience to fit him for the society of which he is a part or to qualify him for a trade or profession. (2:113)

According to Patty,

The Health Education Curriculum is a systematic organization of courses, and of other activities, experiences, and situations which may contribute to the optimal health education development of the pupil. (3:4)

While these definitions are in general agreement, they do differ in that the first two definitions refer to the total body of educative experiences while Patty's definition refers to those experiences that may contribute to the health education development of the pupil. Analysis of Patty's definition reveals the fundamental nature of the health education curriculum. The key words in this definition are *systematic organization; courses; other activities, experiences, situations;* and *optimal health education development.*

Before going into an analysis of the nature of the health education curriculum, let us examine two concepts of curriculum, the *vertical curriculum* and the *horizontal curriculum.* Good also defined curriculum as "A systematic group courses or sequence of subjects required for graduation or certification in a major field of study. . . ." (2:113) This definition emphasized the sequence of subjects continuing through the school life of the pupil. This is the concept of *vertical curriculum.* Such a definition, applied to health education, refers to the health education courses taken from year to year that are required or elected for graduation or for professional preparation.

According to Patty's definition there are many activities, experiences, and situations outside the formal instruction program provided in the courses that may contribute to the health education curriculum. This, for any grade level or at any given time, may be described as the *horizontal curriculum.* It cuts across a wide area of pupil experiences at any given time (Figure 6). Perhaps no other area of the school program embraces such a wide variety of experiences as the health education curriculum. These experiences are so wide and so varied in nature as to call on many school disciplines and to involve many types of school personnel. This is the unique feature of the health education curriculum and the one that mandates continuous curriculum planning. It creates something of a dilemma in that it involves many kinds of people with a variety of professional skills, yet at the same time it requires a specialist in the program, an individual with a broad

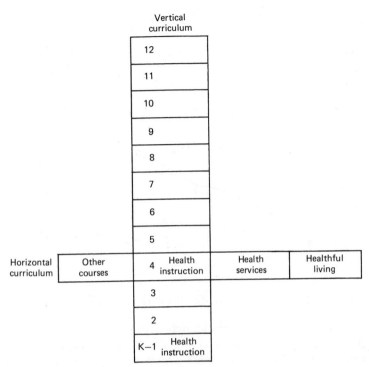

Figure 6. Relationship of the Horizontal and Vertical Health Education Curriculum.

understanding of the health sciences and of human behavior. In all probability, this dilemma helps explain why the need for the health education specialist and for the health education course is often overlooked. With the failure to recognize this need comes the resulting feeling that since everyone is a health teacher there can be no need for the health course or the health teacher. If, as many authorities believe, both kinds of experiences in the educational experiences of the pupil are needed, then it becomes necessary to plan so as to make this possible, incorporating into the curriculum those desirable experiences that will promote the optimum health education development of the pupils.

Components of the Health Education Curriculum

What, then, constitutes the health education curriculum? As mentioned in Chapter 7, the health education curriculum consists of four major components or areas: healthful environment (living), health services, health instruction, and related subjects. The relative contributions made to health education by each of the components, by grade level, is illustrated in Figure 7.

103

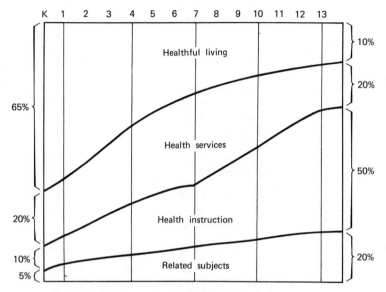

Figure 7. Components of the Health Education Curriculum.

As illustrated in Figure 7, in the kindergarten and grade 1 (K-1) healthful living probably makes the greatest contribution to the health education curriculum. It comprises some 65 percent of the total, with health services amounting to about 20 percent, health instruction 10 percent, and related subjects contributing some 5 percent. At the upper grade levels, grades 10 to 13, the situation is quite different. The contribution of healthful living is probably about 10 percent, health services 20 percent, health instruction 50 percent, and related subjects 20 percent. These data are the composite estimates of several hundred graduate students in health education and are intended to be only rough estimates of the contribution made to the health education of students by each component of the health education curriculum.

Health education aspects of the healthful school environment (healthful living), the day-to-day experiences of the pupil as they relate to the hygienic environment, a hygienic regimen, the school lunch program, and interpersonal relationships, provide important learning experiences. These experiences continue throughout the entire school life of the pupil. By proper planning and through concerted effort they can take their place among the other experiences that are systematically organized to contribute to the optimum health education development of the pupil.

Health education aspects of school health services, the educational possibilities in and through the health service program, are numerous and significant. In fact, the health service program is primarily educational in nature. It should be

104

directed primarily toward preparing students for living in the society in which they find themselves from day to day. In its simplest form the health service program consists of the teacher observations of the health of students, simple first aid measures such as thorough cleansing of minor wounds and abrasions with soap and water, proper protection with a sterile bandage, vision screening, and immunizations. At other times the physical and medical examinations provide unique opportunities for health instruction. The selection and use of community health resources such as the physician or the dentist, assisted and supported by the counsel of the school nurse or medical consultant, helps prepare the students for their role as adults. The extent to which the health service experiences of the pupil are planned and directed toward the education of the pupil determines how much this phase of the program contributes to the health education curriculum. The health service experiences cut across all grade levels. It is important that these experiences be planned to be educational experiences.

Direct health instruction is represented by the health education course of study. This may consist of health units or problems in the early elementary grades or health classes in the higher years, including the secondary school and the college. The health courses may be considered to be the heart of the health education curriculum. They provide the opportunity for acquiring new knowledge, attitudes, and practices, for discarding the unhealthful and strengthening the healthful attitudes and practices, and for integrating the various health education experiences of the individual into a healthful behavioral pattern.

Health instruction in related subjects may be done through correlated teaching (sometimes erroneously called integration), the integrated program, or incidental instruction. *Correlation is a method.* It is the method by which a relationship is shown between another subject to problem area *and* the subject at hand. To illustrate, when the history teacher shows the relationship of the conquest of yellow fever to the success in building the Panama Canal, that teacher is providing health instruction through correlation. The amount of detail included and the time devoted determine whether this procedure becomes direct health instruction. If it involves the full attention of the class, lasting for more than one or two class periods, it moves out of the realm of correlation into direct health instruction. Some areas in which there may be expected to be a considerable amount of health teaching through correlation include biology, general science, chemistry, social science, home economics, and physical education (Chapter 17).

The integrated curriculum also provides numerous opportunities for health instruction. Under this plan there are no courses as such. All teaching is in relation to broad areas or problems (Chapter 17).

Similarly, a considerable amount of health knowledge and attitudes, and some health practices, may be learned as the result of experiences in other courses where there is little or no reference to health. Such learning is the result of inci-

105

dental instruction. Incidental health learning is also a common result of the influence of the healthful, or unhealthful, environment.

The significance of the key words, *systematic organization, courses, activities, experiences,* and *situations* should be noted. It is important to understand that not everything that happens to a child in his school life is a part of the curriculum. This concept of curriculum includes only experiences that are systematically organized and planned as part of the school program. It is usually in written form. This does not preclude the use of unusual and unplanned experiences that may contribute to health education development, but it does recognize that they are not planned experiences and, since they are not likely to happen again by chance, they are not considered a part of the health education curriculum.

The concept of *courses* is well understood, but it should be emphasized that there is need for coordination with other instruction at any given time and articulation with what has been taught and what is planned for future classes or courses. *Activities* may include physical education, intramurals, interscholastics, all kinds of clubs, and field trips as long as there is a planned attempt to contribute to health education development, not just to health. *Experiences* that may constitute a part of the health education curriculum include such things as the teacher screening of weight, height, posture, vision, hearing, and signs of illness; medical and dental examinations; first aid planning and execution; school feeding; committee work such as the student health committee; and education campaign and fund raising for worthy causes. *Situations* that may be systematically organized to promote health education development include the hygienic environment, the sanitary plant, aesthetic surroundings, pleasant teacher-pupil relationships, properly fitting and properly adjusted seats and desks. The mere existence of any facility does not ensure the desired results. Planned situations with appropriate teaching is necessary.

The goal of the health education experiences in this instance is visualized as the *optimum health education development of the pupils.* It is significant that this goal allows for differences in levels of achievement. What may be optimum for one might be beyond the realm of the possible for others or be considerablly below the level of optimum for still others. It is worthy of emphasis that health education is a highly personalized kind of education, geared to meeting the needs of the individual.

The broad and inclusive scope of the health education curriculum can more readily be recognized if it is compared with some of the other curricular areas of the school. What other instructional area calls on so many of the different programs of the school to make up that curriculum? Some other instructional areas do depend to some extent on several different aspects of the school program. Prominent among these would be language arts and social studies, but few, if any, cut across the total school program to the same extent that health education does.

Even though many persons and many programs do contribute to the health education curriculum, *the course of study and the direct instruction that it represents still constitutes the heart of the health education curriculum.* The direct health instruction (course of study) may be likened to the *keystone in an arch.* It is what gives the arch the stability, completing the structure. So it can be with the course of study. It can be the keystone that gives the other health education experiences form and meaning, enabling the pupil to integrate his diverse experiences into a well-rounded personality that has physical, social, emotional, and spiritual dimensions.

This does not minimize the importance of correlation as a method of teaching. Rather, it brings it into focus in its rightful place. In many instances it is the most effective method. However, since by definition it cannot allow the focus of that course to be on health education, there needs to be a series of systematically organized experiences in which the focus is on health education. This is represented by the health education course of study, providing guidance for the course that is intended to facilitate integration of the many health education experiences of the pupil.

Summary

If the goal of health education is to be achieved, the curriculum must be designed to promote that integration of learning within each individual that will tranform knowledge into attitudes resulting in healthful behavior. Such a curriculum cannot be confined to the walls of the health education classroom. It is the responsibility of the school to provide opportunities so that those learning experiences that will facilitate such integration will arise. The systematic organization of courses and of other activities, experiences, and situations can facilitate that kind of integration within the pupil. This is the purpose of the health education curriculum.

References

1. Beauchamp, G.A., *Curriculum Theory*, Third Edition, Kagg, Willmette, Illinois, 1975.
2. Good, C.V., Editor, *Dictionary of Education*, McGraw-Hill, New York, 1959.
3. Patty, W.W., *Syllabus of a Course in Health Education Curriculum*, Indiana University, Bloomington, Indiana, (Out of print).
4. Smith, B.O., W.O. Stanley, and J.H. Shores, *Fundamentals of Curriculum Development*, Revised Edition, World, Yonkers-on-Hudson, 1957.

Chapter Ten
Scheduling and Sequence of Health Instruction

We have proposed that decisions regarding the health education curriculum should be made at three levels: first, the broad general decisions that need to be made at the community level and that are advisory in nature; second, decisions that are usually made at the administration level (school board and administrators); and third, decisions that are largely the responsibility of teachers, both in preparation of the unit plans and in the classroom.

The three broad approaches to organizing the curriculum that were stated by Oberteuffer et at. (11:76–105) are discussed elsewhere in this textbook (Chapter 12). The specific course is discussed in Chapter 11 while correlation and integration are discussed in Chapter 15. In addition, we have placed great emphasis on the opportunities for health education through health services, healthful living, and other courses. Each of these provides opportunities for one or more of the approaches suggested by Oberteuffer et al. It is noteworthy that the approaches we are suggesting do not conflict with the approaches suggested by Oberteuffer et al., nor do they confine health instruction to the classroom, not even to the school. Rather, wide use must be made of community resources if the health education needs of the students are to be satisfied.

Other plans for organizing the curriculum have been and will be proposed, but within most of them there will be opportunity for one or more of the plans discussed here. There are at least three schools of thought concerning the scheduling and sequence of health instruction. First, and perhaps the most prevalent, there are those who feel that there should be *continuous emphasis* on certain im-

---

* This chapter is based on an article by Rash which was published in *The Journal of School Health*, 24, 5 (1954). Used with the permission of The American School Health Association.

portant health problems. Proponents of the plan, which we shall call the *continuous emphasis* plan, argue that there is so much to teach and so little time in which to teach it that the most important health problems must be considered every year. They reason that since one of the major objectives of health education is the establishing of desirable habits, and since, because of the nature of habits, they can only be established through repeated exercise, it follows that continuous emphasis must be placed on those habits that are being encouraged.

The second school of though proposes that the psychological approach be used and that emphasis be placed on a particular health problem when the opportunity offers itself. Proponents of this plan, which we shall call the *opportunistic plan*, argue that readiness is a vital factor in successful teaching or learning, and that the readiness which is the result of an actual problem or situation provides the ideal opportunity for successful teaching. Using this plan, the teacher takes advantage of the opportunity to teach for health when that opportunity arises.

The third school of thought proposes the *cycle plan*, in which certain health problems are singled out for intensive study or emphasis in a particular year with different problems being given consideration in the two or three succeeding years. Under this plan each of the major health problems, or problem areas, receives special attention every few years. In the meantime there is opportunity to reinforce previous learnings as the need arises. Proponents of the cycle plan argue that this plan makes it possible to give adequate emphasis to the major problem areas on the basis of the changing needs, interests, and abilities of the growing child without the dangers of repetition that are so commonly associated with the continuous emphasis plan and without the dangers of omission that may occur in the opportunistic plan.

In this discussion we are speaking of *direct health instruction* as defined by the Joint Committee (10:7), not indirect, incidental, or concomitant learnings. This point of view does not necessarily presuppose a concentrated health course, since direct health instruction can be provided in other courses and other situations. It is important that health instruction be functional and that there be flexibility to allow for consideration of important health problems.

It should be pointed out that the *continuous emphasis plan* is probably the oldest, and perhaps the most widely used plan even today. In the past the textbook series have tended toward this plan, but it must not be assumed that all plans that are not labeled otherwise are continuous emphasis plans. A textbook series may incorporate the cycle plan, the continuous emphasis plan, or other approaches. There is considerable variation in the subject matter presented at a particular grade level by the textbooks of the different health education series or publishers. This means that when a student changes schools, or when a school changes series, or where textbooks of different series are used in different grade levels of a particular school, there is considerable danger of duplication and/or omission of subject matter.

In defense of the continuous emphasis plan, it may be pointed out that repeated emphasis on a particular health problem or problem area does not necessarily mean duplication of subject matter or experiences. If, and when, the three commonly accepted criteria of need, interest, and comprehension ability form the basis for selecting the desired outcomes to be stressed, it is possible to follow the continuous emphasis plan without duplication. However, there is a serious danger that students get the impression they have been getting the same thing over and over from year to year.

The *psychological approach,* or the opportunistic plan, undoubtedly has had widest application in the kindergarten and first grade. In each succeeding year following the first grade, there is a tendency to move away from this plan. However, the many exciting innovations in schools today increase the opportunities for effective use of this plan. Hass (7:339–340) listed 37 innovations and trends in education for transescents (these approaching or just entering adolescence) and early adolescents that are worthy of investigation.

In an effort to capitalize on the merits of both the continuous emphasis plan and the psychological approach, and to eliminate the apparent repetition resulting from unwise use of the continuous emphasis plan, the cycle plan was devised. As indicated in Chapter 1, it was first published in the 1933 Tentative Course of Study in Physical and Health Education for the Elementary Schools of the State of Indiana. (16) A four cycle plan was also proposed for the public schools of the State of Oregon (8:223–224) in 1945.

The unique feature of the cycle or spiral plan is the indepth study of a few selected problem areas each year over a period of some three years or until the major health problem areas have been studied in depth, at which time a new cycle is started in which the same problem areas are again considered at a higher level. For example, a problem that was studied in grade four might again be considered in grades seven and ten.

Within each of the plans the criteria for selecting the expected outcomes remain the same: need, interests, comprehension ability, dependency, and community values. When these criteria are given proper consideration in the planning, other factors that influence the planning of the curriculum fall into line and the primary focus remains on the welfare of the student. Also, as Russell pointed out, there are vast untapped resources to "add feeling, informational and experience dimensions to classroom learning experiences." (12:189)

While the first cycle plans were quite rigid, a considerable flexibility was soon developed. Some problem areas, such as safety in the lower grades, might be considered more frequently than once every three years and other problem areas less frequently. This modified cycle plan appears to have wide application in the variety of approaches in use today. For example, in the School Health Education Study the importance of levels of progression in teaching toward a concept is emphasized. At each level the behavioral objectives reflect progression and sequence, leading to the development of the concept. The plan allows for use of the cycle, or spiral, plan either in a rather strict sense or modified as the occasion warrants.

In describing the vertical organization of the health education curriculum, Fodor and Dalis indicated that the organizing elements, such as nutrition or personal health, "are dealt with at each maturity level with increasing complexity." (5:111) Since the maturity levels mentioned correspond to the major grade levels (primary, etc.), this reflects one of the basic concepts of the cycle plan.

A modified cycle plan is also incorporated into the Framework for Health Instruction in California Public Schools (3:4, 7) as evidenced in the designation of the educational level for which certain concepts are appropriate. For example, under Drug Use and Misuse Concept I (when used properly, drugs are beneficial to mankind) is designated for primary and intermediate, Concept II (many factors influence the misuse of drugs) is designated for all grade levels, and Concepts III and IV are each designated for primary and senior high.

Since 1957 the courses of study in health education for the State of Indiana have suggested a *modified cycle plan* consisting of a combination of the cycle plan and the continuous emphasis plan. In certain problem areas, notably personal hygiene, the cycle plan is suggested while in other areas, notably nutrition, the continuous emphasis plan is suggested. The state law in Indiana requires instruction concerning the effects of alcohol and tobacco in grades four through eight, so that the continuous emphasis plan will of necessity operate in these areas during those years.

Criticisms of the Plans

So far in this discussion, we have examined three plans for handling the sequence of health instruction. Let us now look at some of the shortcomings or limitations of the plans.

We have already implied that one of the chief criticisms of the *continuous emphasis plan* is that it encourages repetition or gives the student the impression that there is repetition. We have all heard reports of that expression, "What, health education again?" or "We have had that every year!"

Perhaps a more genuine criticism is that this plan often fails, or the teachers fail, to discriminate between the essential and the nonessential. It too often encourages emphasis on inconsequential outcomes. Of course, this shortcoming is directly associated with a lack of planning, which might be termed a third weakness of the continuous emphasis plan.

The most serious criticism of the *opportunistic plan* seems to be that this plan fails to provide the assurance that each child will have the opportunity to develop the desirable habits, attitudes, and knowledges that experience has shown to be essential. If *the situation* is to be the springboard, we must recognize that some situations just do not always occur; hence, there is no assurance that the important outcomes will be realized. Furthermore, there will be teachers who do not take advantage of the obvious opportunities presented by the teachable moments.

A second serious criticism of the opportunistic plan is that there will be a tendency for an enthusiastic teacher to want to do the whole job. This may interfere with other matters that are important at that particular grade level. However, what seems to be equally important is that teachers, in the higher grades particularly, would be unsure that the lessons they plan will be needed.

A third criticism of the opportunistic plan stems from a recognized strong point or value—that of student participation in the planning. In spite of its recognized value student planning, when carried to the extreme, tends to operate on the assumption that students are better judges of their present and future needs than are adults who have been through those experiences and who may, per chance, have spent the greater part of their lives trying to discover the solutions to the most important problems.

When supporters of the opportunistic plan extol the values of seizing the opportunity for a health lesson in the appearance of that first cold, two questions seem appropriate: Why wait for that first cold when it might be prevented; and what assurance is there that it will always appear? It would also be appropriate to inquire how such a lesson fits into the long range plan of all of the teachers. Is it not possible that the appearance of that first cold in each classroom will be the stimulus to a unit on colds every year of the child's school life? If these conditions exist the opportunistic plan might easily lead to more repetition than does the traditional "continuous emphasis" plan.

Now, let's be critical of the *cycle plan*. There are two criticisms. First, the cycle plan does not make it possible to take full advantage of the experiences and situations that may arise. There may be occasions when the teacher deliberately avoids taking full advantage of a situation because the problem at hand is scheduled for intensive consideration at another time. Second, the cycle plan does not provide for the continuous emphasis that seems essential for the development of certain habits.

Each of the plans has its strengths and weaknesses. Furthermore, no single plan will prove satisfactory all of the time. Since the modified cycle plan seems to allow for taking advantage of the strengths of each of the other plans, while at the same time avoiding some of the weaknesses, it merits special consideration.

Scheduling of Health Instruction

How should the health instruction be scheduled? Health education classes are generally confined to secondary schools, and we need not speculate much concerning the solution. Dr. Kilander (9:149–159) and his committee gave some clues

113

to the answer in the article, "Health Education as a College Entrance Unit." Briefly, the acceptance of health education credit as a college entrance unit was in direct relationship to the length and intensity of the course. In other words, health education units earned in courses meeting daily for a full year for one full credit were found to have widest acceptance; those earned in courses meeting daily for a semester for one-half unit had the next widest acceptance; those earned by accumulating credit over two or more years on the basis of one, two, or three hours per week were next in acceptance; and those earned when health education was combined with physical education were least accepted as college entrance credits. With the increasing recognition of health education as a distinct discipline, as evidenced by the state certification requirements as reported by Castile and Jerrick (4), the problem of credit should be minimized. Also, with the introduction of flexible scheduling, block time, and learning through discovery, to mention a few of the recent innovations, the most important consideration is the place given health education in the school curriculum.

The pattern of scheduling of health instruction in elementary schools cannot be reduced to classes. There will be occasions for classes in the upper elementary grades, for special health education units at any or all levels, for correlated instruction at all levels, and for the integrated program in the lower grades at least. Provision should be made for independent study, block time scheduling, laboratory periods, field trips, flexible scheduling, and ability achievement. The specific scheduling pattern for a given situation is determined by decisions that must be made locally. The important consideration is that health education has the same status as other courses.

Selecting Health Problem Areas for Consideration

As has been indicated, when the curriculum committee, or subcommittee, is guided by the suggested criteria for selecting expected outcomes and related content, the specific problem areas to be considered will be a logical outgrowth of committee deliberations. The criterion of need will usually be the most important consideration in selecting the outcomes to be desired. At the same time, appropriate consideration must be given to student interests, comprehension ability, dependency, and community values in line with the expressed philosophy of the school and community.

In order to provide a point of reference regarding the health problem areas that have been found to need consideration, the following list of problem areas with their common subproblem areas is suggested. The list is not intended to be exhaustive or directive. Curriculum planners will find other areas that are more important in their particular situations, and some of them will be rejected. The grade placement of the problem areas may vary from place to place depending on the judgment of the committee and the application of the criteria in the local situation.

some common health problem areas

Community and Environmental Health: *Community health problems, ecology, international health.*

Consumer Health: *Advertising, health careers, health insurance, official health agencies, quackery, selecting health services, voluntary health agencies.*

Dental Health: *Care of teeth, dental services, diet, fluoridation.*

Diseases: *Acute noncommunicable, chronic, communicable, deficiency.*

Emotional Health: *Aging (Gerontology), death, stress, self-concept, interpersonal relations, peer group pressures, values.*

Family Living and Parenthood: *Dating, selecting a mate, human sexuality, marriage, parenthood, contraception, family relationships, heredity and environment.*

Mood Modifiers: *Amphetamines, barbiturates, hallucinogens, narcotics, stimulants (caffeine, etc.) C.N.S. depressants (alcohol, aspirin, miltown, methaqualene), smoking, habit formation.*

Nutrition and Physical Fitness: *Diet, exercise, personal health practices, weight control.*

Safety: *Bicycle safety, first aid, highway safety, industrial safety, pedestrian safety, safety in the home.*

Individuals desiring an extensive listing of health content or problem areas may wish to refer to the article by Hardt which appeared in the January, 1978 issue of *The Journal of School Health.* (6)

The conceptual approaches used in the School Health Education Study (13:20) provide another approach in organizing instructional materials. The writing team selected 10 major concepts toward which the instructional materials are to be directed. Within the framework of each of these concepts, long range goals are suggested in each domain, and subconcepts and behavioral objectives are suggested for each progression level.

Whereas the School Health Education Study writing team proceeded from the major concepts to subconcepts and behavioral objectives, the Commission on Curriculum Development of the AAHPER (1) selected major problem areas and proceeded to develop concepts within these areas. Another approach in selecting health problem areas for consideration was used in developing the Bureau of Health Education's Elementary School Health Education Curriculum Project (Berkeley Model). (2) The program uses the unit plan involving a comprehensive health education approach organized around a body system. Stress is placed on how individual behavior and interaction with the environment impacts on the body system.

One of the outstanding features of the program is the training of a *team* of four or five persons responsible for introducing the program into a school. After

115

the program has been demonstrated in the school by the team, it is then expanded to others in that school.

The health education program in the State of New York is organized along what they call the Strand approach. They selected *optimal health* as the goal to be achieved through knowledge, attitudes, and behavior. To achieve this goal they selected the five major strands or problem areas: physical health, sociological health problems, mental health, environmental and community health, and education for survival. Each of these strands includes appropriate subproblem areas. (14: 81–87).

Summary

It is vitally important that health instruction be on the same basis as other important instruction. As far as scheduling is concerned, this will vary from grade to grade. It seems logical and desirable to require a full unit of credit in the junior high school based on a course that meets daily for a full year, or the equivalent in block time scheduling, and another full unit in the senior high school on an elective basis.

In the past we have emphasized the commonly accepted criteria of *need, interest,* and *comprehension ability* as the basis for selecting expected outcomes. To these criteria two others should be added, *community values* and *dependency.* In actual practice it is not unusual to recognize quietly the importance of community attitudes in relation to instruction in the controversial areas. It is time to become realistic and recognize community values as another criterion by which we are guided in our selection of expected outcomes and content. The criterion of dependency is an important consideration in planning for health education. In simple terms it can be expressed as *emphasize that which the child can do something about by himself.* In the light of this criterion, it follows that cleanliness will occupy an important place during the early grades while certain emphases on nutrition, such as planning the diet, may need to be reserved until the student is more nearly self-supporting. It is evident that certain aspects of family life education are appropriate in the junior high school, and that instruction concerning drugs, including tobacco and alcohol, should precede the time when there is a tendency to begin their use.

Since it is obviously impossible to make specific recommendations concerning all areas, let us consider the possible contribution of a coordinating committee headed by a person who has the responsibility of coordinating efforts and articulating instruction. The title of health coordinator is appropriate for someone doing this kind of work (Chapter 4).

The exact nature of the coordinating committee will vary from place to place. However, in each instance its primary function will be to serve as a clear-

116

inghouse for ideas, opportunities, and responsibilities that will facilitate the health education program (Chapter 6).

When the health education curriculum committee of a school arrives at an allocation of responsibilities to the various grade levels on the basis of the accepted criteria, we need not worry too much about what plan to follow. Such an approach is very likely to result in something of a modified cycle plan. However, the particular plan is not important.

What is important is that there will be conscious planning at the local level on the basis of the criteria of need, interest, comprehension ability, dependency, and community values. There must be sufficient flexibility to allow for continuous emphasis when necessary, for use of the psychological approach when appropriate, and for a cycle plan when it seems desirable.

In reality, the solution of the problem of scheduling and sequences rests not so much in a particular plan as it does with the planners.

References

1. American Association for Health, Physical Education, and Recreation, *Health Concepts: Guides for Health Instruction*, AAHPER, Washington, D.C., 1967.

2. Bureau of Health Education, *Focal Points*, Center for Disease Control, Atlanta, Georgia, February, 1976.

3. California State Department of Education, *Framework for Health Instruction in California Public Schools, Kindergarten Through Grade Twelve*, California State Department of Education, Sacramento, 1970.

4. Castile, A.S. and S.J. Jerrick, "School Health in America: A Summary Report of a Survey of the State School Health Programs," *The Journal of School Health*, 46: 4 (1976).

5. Fodor, J.T. and G.T. Dalis, *Health Instruction: Theory and Application*, Lea & Febiger, Philadelphia, 1966.

6. Hardt, D.V., "Health Curriculum: 370 Topics," *The Journal of School Health*, 48, 656–660 (1978).

7. Hass, G., "Education for Transescents and Early Adolescents," *Curriculum Planning, A New Approach*, Allyn, 1977.

8. Hoyman, H.S., "Oregon's Four-Cycle Health Curriculum," *Journal of School Health and Physical Education*, 18: 4 (1947).

9. Kilander, H.F., "Health as a College Entrance Unit," *The Journal of School Health*, 21: 5 (1951).

10. Moss, B.R., Editor, *Health Education*, N.E.A., Washington, D.C., 1961.

11. Oberteuffer, D., O.A. Harrelson, and M.B. Pollock, *School Health Education*, Harper & Row, 1972.

117

12. Russell, R.D., *Health Education*, Project of the Joint Committee on Health Problems in Education of the N.E.A. and the A.M.A., National Education Association, Washington, D.C., 1975.

13. School Health Education Study, *Health Education: A Conceptual Approach to Curriculum Design*, School Health Education Study, Washington, D.C., 1967.

14. Sinacore, John, "New York State's Program in the Health Sciences," *The Bulletin of the National Association of Secondary School Principals*, 52: 326 (1968).

15. "Special Issue: Design and Implementation of School Health Curricula," *Journal of School Health* 48: 4 (1978).

16. State of Indiana, *Tentative Course of Study in Physical and Health Education*, Grades One to Eight, State Department of Public Instruction, Indianapolis, 1933.

Chapter Eleven
The Course of Study in Health Education

The health education curriculum of a school or school system includes the written plans for making the school health program an educational program. It should deal with all four aspects of the program and should contain in some detail the plans for making the experiences educational. As one of the four major components of the health education curriculum, and perhaps the most important one, the course of study merits special consideration.

Some recent attempts at evaluating the health instruction program in secondary schools have revealed a general and serious weakness in the planning that should be done for health instruction. The School Health Education Study revealed "a marked deficiency in the quantity and quality of health education in both the elementary and secondary schools." (4) Ludwig and Schaller (2) found the almost complete absence of systematic planning for health instruction at the level of unit and course of study planning. In school health program surveys conducted annually over a period of 25 years, Rash (3) found that the development and use of a course of study was consistently one of the weakest areas of the school health program.

The results of the Indiana School Health Education Study supported the hypothesis that the health education program of the schools studied was failing to motivate students to reach their full potential in health knowledge, attitudes, and practices.

It should be obvious that sound planning is basic to a good educational program. Too often, however, the textbook is accepted as the sole guide, if not the entire content, of the health education course. Although a considerable amount of planning has gone into the preparation of a textbook, such planning cannot take into consideration the particular needs and interests of a specific community. The kind of planning that is essential can only be done at the local level, by persons who are familiar with the situation, and by involving people who are to be taught as well as those who are to do the teaching. This strongly suggests the desirability of developing a guide for the local situation.

Nature of the Course of Study

Any guide that might be developed for a school or school system should consider all aspects of the school health program. It should contain written policies on procedures to be followed in carrying on the school program in a manner that will make it educational and also fulfill the special functions of health services, environmental protection, etc. This will include policies for meeting emergency situations such as fire or tornado, providing emergency care through first aid, routine program activities, public relationships, and individual responsibilities of administrators, teachers, pupils, and parents. It should include organizational arrangements for conduct of the program, areas of responsibility, and lines of authority. Furthermore, it should include plans for promoting a close, smooth working relationship between related departments (coordination).

In addition to unit plans, the course of study should contain introductory and explanatory information that will be helpful to the users. It should include statements of the basic philosophy of the group developing the course of study. Such statements serve as general guides for the users as well as revealing some of the reasons underlying the particular selection of materials in the course of study. For example, a statement pointing out why sex education is considered important will assist the teacher in planning the instruction in this area. A statement that firmly establishes the place of health education as an important, academically respectable discipline meriting consideration equal to that given other academically respectable areas would provide some degree of motivation and security for the health educators. Furthermore, it is vitally important that the unity of the school health and the public health program be firmly established, as discussed in Chapters 5 and 6.

If, as we have indicated earlier, school health is public health in a special place, it is incumbent upon school health educators to take the initiative in promoting the unity of the total community health program. The community health educator, or coordinator, and other public health personnel should be involved in planning the school health program so that it will make the greatest possible contribution to the total community program. Those charged with the responsibility of developing the instructional units, whether for use by teachers, physicians, nurses, environmental health or administrative personnel, should make certain that plans include wide use of community resources. If students are to understand, use, and support worthy community health programs, it is important that they be given those opportunities throughout their school life.

In the total framework of the health education curriculum the *course of study* is, without doubt, the most important consideration. While it is important to recognize the contributions made to the health education of students by health services, the healthful environment, and other aspects of the school program, the *course,* as represented by the course of study, constitutes the heart of the total educational program.

From the beginning of the project it should be recognized that the development of a course of study, from initial planning to distribution, is a *three year project,* even when released time is allowed for key committee personnel. This time schedule should be kept in mind in making appointments to committees and in assigning special responsibilities. It is also an important consideration in relation to the revision of the course of study.

In addition to some statements of philosophy the introduction should deal with such aspects of the curriculum as time allotment, grade placement, credit, preparation outside of class (including homework), relationship to other departments, joint use of facilities and equipment by several departments, the role of the parents in a successful health education program, and other matters that may influence the conduct of the program.

The Course of Study Defined

The course of study *is an official guide prepared for use by teachers, supervisors, administrators, and others with responsibilities for health education.* It is systematically organized by units of instruction for the designated grades with expected outcomes; content; methods, devices, and techniques (instructional media); supplies and equipment; references; and suggested procedures for evaluating the success in attaining the expected outcomes through the direct instruction.

The Suggestive Nature of the Course of Study

There are differences of opinion, and in practice, concerning the extent to which the course of study is suggestive or directive. In most instances a course of study is *suggestive* of areas and topics that may be included in the instruction. This is generally true for a statewide course of study which may serve as a guide and resource for developing local plans. However, as the local level is approached there might be increasing justification for a more directive approach, especially if there appeared to be a need for uniformity in the content of different courses in the same school or school system. However it would be a rare instance when the course of study would be literally a directive of the content of the course. Indeed this would be contrary to one of the basic criteria for planning the health education program, the criterion of *need.* It is most important that the needs of each student be given consideration.

121

Within areas or topics the selection of expected outcomes to be stressed will, of necessity, vary from group to group and from individual to individual. The variation will be so great as to make the teaching of questionable value, if not completely ineffective, if the expected outcomes to be stressed are preselected or mandated. If it is sound practice to be guided by the criteria (need, interest, comprehension ability, dependence, and community values) in selecting expected outcomes to be stressed, then it follows that the selection must be made in terms of the criteria as they apply to the student(s) at hand.

One word of caution concerning the suggestive nature of the course of study may be appropriate. Deviations from the suggested pattern may be desirable, but any such deviation should not include health education units planned for higher grades. This does not preclude the use of teachable moments, but if an entire unit is taken from a later grade, without agreement of the other teacher, it might easily undermine and destroy the effectiveness of instruction planned for later grades. Any need for such modification of plans should be brought to the attention of the course of study committee for consideration in a revision of the course of study.

The suggestive nature of the course of study is even more significant in regard to the content and the methods, devices, and techniques of instruction. Differences in students, as well as differences in the background and special competencies of the teachers, dictate that a wide variety of content items must be available for use in providing instruction intended to achieve the desired outcomes. Furthermore, a wide choice of approaches will be necessary to cope with the varied interests and abilities of the students, thus necessitating the suggestion of a wide variety of methods, devices, and techniques that might be used. The role of the health coordinator becomes important in this regard, both as a resource person and as the promoter and coordinator of an inservice education program.

The Tentative Nature of the Course of Study

In addition to the nondirective nature of the course of study, it is important to note that it is *tentative* in nature. This point is so important as to suggest that the word, tentative, be used in the title of the publication. It is a serious mistake to allow anyone to assume that a course of study is of a permanent nature. Constant evaluation and frequent revision of even the most up-to-date and progressive course of study is an absolute necessity. No more than five years should elapse before publication of a revised version of any course of study. In actual practice revision should be a continuous, ongoing process. Furthermore, the need for constant revision and the suggestive nature of the course of study indicate the desirability of updating by each person who uses the course of study. Any such revision should be reported to the appropriate committee for use in the next revision of the guide. Except in a strictly local situation, and then on a purely tentative

122

basis, it is not possible to define the exact nature of the instruction needed to meet the varied and changing health education needs in the world today.

The specific content of the course of study will vary from situation to situation, but the general form may remain fairly constant. The unit plans make up the major content of the course of study. Procedures for developing the unit plan are explained elsewhere. Suffice it to say, the essential elements in the unit are: title; expected outcomes; content; methods, devices, and techniques; teaching aids; evaluation procedures; and references. These need not appear in this exact form, but they are all essential to the adequate unit.

Cooperative Development of the Course of Study

It is a fact or principle not generally recognized that the greatest value of the curriculum project, including the development of the course of study, comes to those who participate in its development. This principle has long been recognized in successful voluntary agency work, as well as in business.

Many factors, such as the pressure of time and other essential extracurricular responsibilities, seem to contribute to a tendency among school administrators to involve as few people as possible in any particular project. Such a practice, if followed in a course-of-study development, immediately precludes reaping the greatest benefits of the project by the greatest number of people.

Since the course of study will be developed jointly, involving several people, it is a good policy to give credit to those who participate in its development. This can be done by appropriate acknowledgements, either in the introduction or in the appendix.

Editing and Publishing the Course of Study

The editing and publishing of the course of study is the responsibility of the central course of study committee. It will ordinarily work through delegated committees, but the final responsibility for publication rests with this committee.

The first step is reading and checking the copy for absolute accuracy in every respect. This needs to be done by selected members of the course of study committee, those selected for their special abilities in performing this function. In addition to their knowledge of health and health education, they must be adept at proofreading.

The second step involves editing for logical arrangement, ease of reading, effective presentation, and other factors that might influence the effectiveness of the course of study. Special attention should be given to ensure that the introduction, or the foreword, provides the essential general explanatory information that will facilitate the use of the guide. The acknowledgments should include all who served on any committee, the tryout personnel, persons or organizations pro-

123

viding special information or materials, and recognition to authors or publishers of copyrighted material used by permission.

The third step, the actual printing, involves decisions regarding the medium of printing and the binding or cover to be used. It may be reproduced in one of several forms such as ditto, mimeograph, xerox, or printing. If the project is strictly for local use or for tryout on a wider basis, the mimeograph or the xerox is satisfactory. If the course of study is prepared for wider distribution, after an initial tryout and revision, printing is more desirable. A printed cover is often desirable even though the body of the publication is mimeographed. The binding of the document may be either in loose-leaf or permanent form. The main advantage of loose-leaf binding is that sections of the course of study may be replaced with the revised version. The permanent binding, stapled or stitched, is less expensive and somewhat more durable than loose-leaf binding. The front cover should provide for a title, the statement of grades included, the identification of the school system, and the date of publication. The title would ordinarily be "A Tentative Course of Study in Health Education," the word "tentative" suggesting the evolutionary nature of the good course of study.

Additional desirable features of the course of study include a foreword, acknowledgments, explanatory statements, special recognition of copyright holders for material quoted, and other explanatory statements. Regular documentation procedures should be followed. A table of contents facilitates the use of the course of study. There should be a general introduction to the course of study. The introduction may present some of the philosophy of the parent body as well as provide other information that may have some relation to the use of the course of study. Short introductory statements may precede the various sections of the course of study.

There are some advantages to binding the course of study by individual grades, such as focusing attention of the teacher on the grade concerned and economy. However, binding by combinations of grades for lower elementary, upper elementary, and secondary school would provide the advantage of advising the teacher of what has gone before and what is to follow, thus promoting articulation between grade levels.

Distributing the Course of Study

To give the proper emphasis to the significance of completion of the course of study project and to give due recognition to those who participated, it is desirable to arrange for a rather formal presentation of the finished product to the health education curriculum advisory council and to the superintendent of schools and his staff. However, the most important and most difficult task is that of placing the course of study into the hands of every teacher, supervisor, administrator, and other health education person who has responsibility for health education.

Key citizens should not be overlooked in the distribution. No set formula for distribution can be proposed. However, a systematic mailing, distribution at conferences and institutes, and a continuous vigil for persons who have not received a copy will pay dividends through improved instruction. Any mailing of courses of study should be by the personal name of the recipient. No effort should be spared to avoid the accumulation of unused courses of study on some bookshelf.

It may appear to be a relatively simple plan to mail, or otherwise deliver, a copy of the printed course of study to each administrator and health teacher in the school system, but this becomes increasingly complex and difficult as the size of the system increases. On a local or a county basis a special committee may be charged with the responsibility for distributing the course of study. On a state-wide basis the distribution can probably be best accomplished by the official agency sponsoring the project. In any case, special plans need to be made to get copies of the publication to the appropriate people on first distribution and then, and more difficult to accomplish, to see that new administrators and new teachers receive copies as soon as they join the system. In all instances, provision must be made to be certain that each individual who possesses a course of study is supplied with any partial revisions as they are prepared. This is a most difficult task, which is complicated by our mobile society with a high turnover rate of teaching personnel.

One of the most important steps in developing the course of study is teacher orientation. Plans must be developed to provide the opportunity for explaining the new course of study to teachers or for briefing teachers on revisions. Some approaches might be through summer workshops or institutes, teachers' meeting at the opening of school, special inservice education meetings early in the school year and periodically thereafter, and credit courses in adult education or extension programs.

Evaluating and Revising the Course of Study

Special provision should always be made for an ongoing program of evaluation and revision of the course of study. This may be done very satisfactorily by appointing a continuing committee to carry on, or promote, such activity. This committee should have as its chairman some person representing the official sponsoring agency who is in position to keep in touch with progress in health and health education and who will be alert to opportunities to improve the course of study as well as to needed revisions. The committee should include representatives of the teachers who are using the guide, the health coordinator or supervisor, and students. The committee members must be cognizant of new developments, both in education and in health.

Evaluation of the total school health education program will be discussed in Chapter 20. Evaluation of the course of study should follow some of the same procedures. However, the primary concerns in this instance center on the adequacy of the guide in assisting teachers. There needs to be a planned system of reporting needed revisions by teachers and students who are using the guide. Specific individuals should be charged with the responsibility of reporting new developments. The committee should meet regularly to assess the situation and make recommendations for implementing the necessary revisions.

Various individual units could be revised without attempting to revise the entire course of study, particularly if it is in loose-leaf binders. The problem of distributing revised units to persons having the course of study is difficult to handle, but this can be approached through keeping systematic records of persons who received the course of study. There will, inevitably, be some who cannot be reached, but by giving wide publicity to the revision most interested persons can be informed.

Whereas courses of study in some areas may be considered appropriate for several years, health education is so closely related to new discoveries in the health sciences and to the changing concepts in the behavioral sciences that a period of a few months sometimes renders certain parts out of date. A constant vigil is necessary and seldom could a course of study in health education be considered up-to-date if it is as much as five years old. Evaluation will be discussed in greater detail in Chapter 20.

Summary

The course of study represents the heart of the health education program, providing assistance in coordinating the health education program and in articulating the health instruction from year to year. Organization for developing the course of study will be included in plans for curriculum development and may follow the appropriate suggestions found under the topic of Organization for Health Education Curriculum Development. The course of study is the direct responsibility of the central course of study committee that should have charge of allocating responsibilities to appropriate committees and persons.

The value of the course of study project will be closely related to the importance attached to it by teachers, course of study committee personnel, and administrators. To enjoy optimum success the project must have the interest and enthusiastic support of all concerned.

References

1. Jones, Herb, Project Director, *Indiana School Health Education Study*, Department of Physiology and Health Science, Ball State University, Muncie, Indiana, 1976.

126

2. Ludwig, D.J., and W.E. Schaller, unpublished report on *A Study of Health Education in Selected Indiana Secondary Schools*, Indiana University, Bloomington, Indiana, 1965.

3. Rash, J.K., unpublished reports of *School Health Surveys*, Indiana University, Bloomington, Indiana, 1949–1974.

4. Sliepcevich, E.M., *School Health Education: A Call for Action!* School Health Education Study, Washington, D.C., 1965.

Chapter Twelve
Planning the Health Education Unit

Direct health instruction has a prominent role in the total health education curriculum of our schools and colleges of today. Direct instruction, in this instance, refers to that deliberate planned instruction designed to favorably influence habits, attitudes, and knowledges relating to health. It may take place in the health education class or in other classes in which the direct approach may be used.

The health education curriculum has been defined as a "systematic organization of courses and other activities, experiences, and situations which contribute to the optimal health education development of the pupil."(9) Note that this definition of curriculum does not include all that happens to a child or all of his or her experiences. It is recognized that such experiences do have their influence, but this definition of curriculum includes only those activities, experiences, and situations (including courses) that are a part of the systematically organized program of the school.

The course of study is one important aspect of the health education curriculum. It has been defined as *an official guide prepared for use by teachers, supervisors, administrators, and others with a responsibility for health education.* It is specifically concerned with the health instruction program.

Oberteuffer et al. (8:78) suggested several different approaches in teaching health education, including, the separate course, broad fields (correlation), and integration (core curriculum). Past experience and current practice favors the separate course approach. This does not preclude the use of correlation in related courses and/or health instruction in the integrated or core curriculum. In fact,

---

* This chapter is based on an article by Rash that was published in *The Journal of the American Association for Health, Physical Education, and Recreation, 24,* 9, (1953). Used with the permission of the American Alliance for Health, Physical Education, and Recreation.

129

the health course can provide the opportunity to bring together all of the health education experiences and to integrate them into a pattern of healthful behavior.

Some approaches to teaching that were reported by Cauffman (3:158–174) include the use of textbooks, problem solving, lecture and group discussion, and instructional media (audiovisual techniques). Other approaches can be developed by ingenious teachers. The important thing to remember is that good teaching doesn't "just happen." It requires careful planning, and the preparation of a unit plan is one essential step in that process.

Need for Planned Units of Instruction

Regardless of the organization pattern, the plan of scheduling, or the approach in teaching, there needs to be a plan that details the needs to be met (expected outcomes), what to teach to meet those needs, some suggested approaches to teaching (methods, devices, and techniques, including teaching aids), some procedures by which to evaluate the success in attaining the desired expected outcomes, and important references for both the teacher and the pupils. The unit plan provides such a vehicle for meeting those needs.

A unit is a plan for developing selected expected outcomes in a problem area within *a course of study*. The unit plan is intended to provide a written outline of the proposed educational experiences in a particular aspect of health, a health problem, leading to the optimum health education development of the students.

If direct health instruction is to serve its intended purpose, there must be a well-conceived plan to guide the education experiences. This does not preclude the taking advantage of spontaneous situations (teachable moments). However, it does assume that such experiences are not enough to do the whole job in a systematic way, making for certain essential, specific, and measurable outcomes. If desirable outcomes are to be achieved, particularly in teaching that is intended to take advantage of spontaneous situations, teachers must plan for most of the situations that can arise and how they will take advantage of them. This might not call for a full scale unit but if one has been planned it will facilitate instruction.

It is generally agreed by health educators that the *traditional textbook* teaching of the past is woefully inadequate in developing desirable practice outcomes and that it seldom achieves optimum success in developing desirable attitudes. However, until our schools are staffed with teachers who have the necessary scientific health knowledge coupled with the desirable "know-how" of modern educational methods, we must continue to expect textbooks to have a prominent place in the health education classroom. Hopefully they will be used as resources and not as the only source of information.

There are at least two broad general classifications of units: the instruction or teaching unit and the resource unit. While the focus of this presentation is on the instruction unit the same basic procedures will be used in developing the resource unit. The resource unit differs from the instruction unit mainly in that it is broader or more general and because it is adaptable to a wider variety of circumstances. It will usually contain many more expected outcomes and dependent materials and will therefore be longer. While the instruction unit will ordinarily include only those materials that may be expected to be used by most teachers the resource unit includes a wide variety of materials from which the teacher will have to choose according to the criteria applied to those students.

Essential Considerations in Planning the Unit

The basic criteria for selection of the unit, including outcomes that are expected and the subsequent content designed to help the learner develop the desired outcomes, are the same for health education as for other areas of education. It is true that the various criteria may have more weight in one instance than in another, or in one area of knowledge than in another, but generally speaking, the criteria of *need, interest, comprehension ability, dependency,* and *community values* should determine the nature of the program.

The nature of the educational outcomes to be expected in health education, like the criteria previously mentioned, is again common to other areas of education. The nature of the expected outcomes to be stressed may vary from subject to subject, age to age, and community to community; but in any event, educational outcomes will be expressed in terms of *practices* (or *habits*), *attitudes*, and *knowledges*. In short, learners will be influenced and their health conserved to the extent that they are influenced in what they do, feel, or know (Chapter 13).

The stating of educational outcomes in terms of behavior changes, as is emphasized here, is in agreement with the suggestions of Alberty (1), Smith, Stanley, and Shores (12), Hopkins (5), Johns (6), Mager (7), Wood and Lerrigo (14), Tyler (13), and others. Early health educators, such as Thomas D. Wood, M.D. and Jesse Ferring Williams, M.D., also recognized the importance of behavioral outcomes in health education. In this sense they were early pioneers, well ahead of their time in that emphasis.

Planning the Unit

The first step in planning a unit must of necessity be selecting the health problem area to be considered. The area will be selected on the basis of the accepted criteria. As stated previously, the criterion of need will be of prime importance in guiding the selection, but the other criteria must also be considered.

The outline for a unit includes eight major headings, corresponding to the steps necessary in planning the unit. The following outline has been proposed (9):

1. Name or title of unit
2. Long range goals
3. Outcomes expected in the learner. (These will be discussed in detail in Chapter 13.)
4. Content intended to contribute to the achievement of expected outcomes (Chapter 14).
5. Methods, devices, and techniques (instructional media) designed to best present the content (Chapter 16).
6. Teaching aids necessary for making the various methods and devices effective.
7. Evaluation procedures to be used to evaluate pupil achievement of expected outcomes and, of course, effectiveness of teaching.
8. References and materials for the learner and for the teacher.

Various forms may have been proposed for presenting the unit plan, each of which may be satisfactory.

Grout suggested that a unit plan should include:

I. Title of unit, preferably stated in the form of a problem or question.

II. General objectives of unit, stated in terms of student accomplishments.

III. Suggested approaches (how the unit may be introduced.)

IV. Body of unit:

Problems, Interests, and Needs	Specific Objectives	Concepts and Content	Teacher and Pupil Activities (Learning Activities)	Materials

V. Plan for evaluation. (4:151)

Read and Green listed the following "six essential elements of the unit as given by Blount and Klausmeier—I. Introductory Statement. II. Outline of Objectives. III. Content Outline. IV. Learning Activities. V. Materials and Resources. VI. Evaluation Procedures." (10:66–67)

The format for the Teaching-Learning Guide shown in *Health Education, A Conceptual Approach to Curriculum Design*, (11:99) is shown below.

Behavioral Objectives and Content	Teacher and Student Materials	Learning Opportunities	Evaluation Activities

The behavioral outcomes and content are listed together to clarify their relationship. The column headings are self-explanatory.

From the unit plan outlines shown, it will be obvious that, although the format varies the basic content is similar and that special emphasis is placed on the objectives and the content used to attain those objectives. However, the parallel column format has special merit. The basic layout of a unit according to this plan is shown in Figure 8. It has the advantage of making ready reference to preceding items, thus facilitating the development of the unit in the light of all factors to be considered. Using this format, the plans for each expected outcome can be developed on a single sheet of $8^1/_2''$ by $14''$ paper. When the *expected outcome* has been stated the next step is to select and list the appropriate *content*. This will be discussed in Chapter 13. Next comes the selection and listing of appropriate *methods, devices*, and *techniques* for using the selected content to develop the expected outcome. Any special *teaching aids*, such as laboratory supplies and equipment, should be listed in the teaching aids column. These should all be listed for each outcome. Later they may be compiled into lists without duplication from which the teacher may select appropriate methods, devices, and techniques and related teaching aids. *Evaluation procedures* must be selected for their effectiveness in determining whether the expected outcomes were attained. The *references* should be selected in relation to the content to be used. They are listed in the last column for expediency, to allow for flexibility in listing them.

The completed unit may be published in the horizontal format shown in Figure 8 or it may be published in semi-outline form. As a matter of expediency it is often more convenient to use the semi-outline form, since it is easier to type in this form than in the horizontal form. If the outline form is used, care should be exercised to show the relationship between the expected outcome and the related content by numbering them accordingly, for example, content number 1 goes with expected outcome number 1, etc. (See Appendix C.)

name or title of unit

Two considerations are essential in selecting a title for the unit. The title should *inform and motivate*. It must, first of all, convey to the reader a distinct concept of the general nature of the unit. At the same time it should stimulate the reader to want to know more about the subject. The detail of the title may vary, depending in part on the developmental level of the learner. As shown in the Sample Unit for K-1, a safety unit might be titled *Traveling Safely To and From School* as opposed to *School Safety* as a title. The latter might satisfy the needs of the teacher,

Problem Area _____
Title of Unit _____
Long Range Goal _____ Grade _____

Expected Outcomes	Content	Methods, Devices, and Techniques	Teaching Aids	Evaluation Procedures	References Teacher Student
Stated in terms of:					
1. *Knowledge*	Problems, subject matter, information, and/or situations designed to develop the expected outcomes.	Instructional systems, teaching methods, activities, procedures, and/or approaches to be used in teaching the content to achieve the expected outcomes.	Supplies, equipment, materials, and helps of different kinds needed for a particular method, device, or technique.	Instruments, procedures, ways, means, and devices for determining the success in attaining the expected outcomes.	Books, magazines, pamphlets, films, resource materials, etc. to be used as sources of content and/or as guides for methods to be used in attaining the expected outcomes.
2. *Attitudes*					*Teacher References Pupil References*
3. *Practices*	*Relate to Column 1*	*Relate to Column 2*	*Relate to Column 3*	*Relate to Column 1*	*Relate to Columns 1 and 2*

Figure 8. Suggested form for developing the unit in health education.

but it would lack the motivating stimulus helpful to the student who might like to know more about what is to be studied.

long range goal

Long range goals are of prime importance in health education. They are needed to give direction to the curriculum from year to year, especially in the cycle plan where considerable time may elapse between the time a problem area is studied and when it may be studied again. Whereas the expected outcomes in a problem area will change from grade to grade, the long range goal remains the same and serves to encourage articulation of instruction at different grade levels. To cite an example from the K-1 Safety Unit, the long range goal is: Leads an active, vigorous life free from preventable accidents. Such a goal has application at any grade level, but more specific outcomes must be developed if the long range goal is to be achieved.

expected outcomes (also see chapter thirteen)

As mentioned previously, the educational outcomes in health education will be in terms of practices, attitudes, or knowledges. Furthermore, those outcomes to be stressed at a particular grade level or on a particular occasion must be determined in light of the learner's needs, interests, comprehension ability, dependency, and community values.

The reader may note that we do not use the term "objective" in this presentation. That is a deliberate attempt to focus attention on what happens in the learner and to preclude having to differentiate between teacher objectives and student objectives. Of course, it may be argued that the term "expected outcomes" is just a longer way of saying "objectives." However, it will be noted that there is less occasion for the common retort, "whose objectives?" when it is understood that expected outcomes always refer to student objectives.

The form for expressing the expected outcome seems to be a problem for many people. Too often the expected practice or habit outcome of washing hands before meals is expressed "to develop the habit of washing hands before meals," whereas, what is really intended is, "washes hands before meals." Likewise, an expected attitude outcome is often expressed as "to develop the attitude of liking to be clean," when what is really intended is "likes to be clean." Expected knowledge outcomes are more commonly expressed in the appropriate language of "knows" or "understands."

Mager (7) proposed that all statements of expected outcomes (objectives) should have two characteristics. They should clearly communicate the behavior expected and include the evaluation criterion (or criteria) to be used in judging the success of attaining the desired outcome.

While Mager's proposal has considerable merit in that he proposes using words that are subject to few interpretations, if followed to the letter it might tend to discourage consideration of attitude outcomes. There would appear to be few if any such problems with knowledge or practice outcomes. Because of the subjective nature of attitudes and because the influence of attitudes may not be readily revealed in practice it becomes almost impossible to expect an immediate, overt, manifestation of the attitude as it is expressed in practice. However, few if any health educators would question the desirability, in fact the necessity, of teaching for desirable health attitudes.

Patty (9) suggested that in addition to the five accepted criteria, the following procedures (not to be confused with criteria) may also be used in determining expected outcomes to be included in the course of study: analysis of needs of children and adults; pupil expressions of interests; observation of pupil interests; opinions of health educators, health service staff, and parents; study of the practices revealed in other courses of study; and study of research findings. In addition, practicality or feasibility must at times be considered although every effort should be made to keep feasibility from dictating the curriculum. For example, it may not be feasible for a school to have a swimming pool, but swimming can be included in the physical education program through a cooperative relationship with another agency such as the park department.

content (also see chapter fourteen)

The content column, as suggested in Figure 8, may well be a topical outline of subject matter, information, or situations to be used in realizing the desired outcomes as expressed under expected outcomes. One example of the indication of the content designed to help provide the opportunity for developing the practice of washing hands before meals might well be "how to wash hands." Of course the teacher will make certain that proper procedures are taught.

It is a common error to assume that one content item may be expected to provide the basis for realizing several outcomes. In reality, several content items must ordinarily be called upon to ensure the development of a single outcome. The child does not develop the habit of washing hands before meals simply by learning to wash hands. A veriety of content items (information, subject matter, experiences, and situations) must be provided for each outcome if that expected outcome is to be achieved. This suggestion is not intended to contradict Tyler's (13) assumption that most learning experiences produce multiple outcomes. On the contrary, the recognition of the multiple outcome result confirms the belief that health education instructors must focus on the desired outcome and take all possible steps to develop that outcome, using a variety of content and methodology.

Two natural results of this approach will be a greatly reduced number of ex-

136

pected outcomes, and the almost inevitable allocation of materials to certain specific grade levels. This may, or may not, result in something of a cycle plan. However, it should reduce the amount of repetition that seems to be altogether too common from grade to grade.

In selecting content it is imperative that the subject matter, information, experiences, or situations provide opportunities for developing the desired outcomes. In the athletic program coaches agree that boys do not learn to play basketball by just reading about it. However, the successful coach recognizes the value in the right kind of reading but does not make the mistake of substituting reading for long hours of practice. In health education desirable attitudes and practices are not established just by reading about them. Perfection of a desirable attitude or practice, to the point of habituation, requires practice under varying circumstances over an extended period of time.

Attitudes are commonly the result of how people perceive their experiences; with some notable exceptions such as a tragic experience, they develop as a result of repeated experiences. Thus, to strengthen the desirable attitudes and weaken the undesirable ones, repeated experiences are necessary. In health education, this will often require a cooperative approach between the school staff, representatives of community health agencies, and the home.

methods, devices, and techniques (also see chapter eighteen)

When a desired outcome has been chosen and several items of content selected to lead to the expected outcomes, the next step in unit planning is to determine the most appropriate methods, devices, and techniques (instructional systems) for assisting the learner in quest of each of the expected outcomes.

The number of methods, devices, and techniques for each item of content should allow for a variety of approaches. In short, several methods and devices should be provided for each item of content. There will be, of course, a considerable amount of overlapping of methods applied to different content items. Hence, it is even more important that a variety of appropriate methods and devices be suggested in each instance.

Some of the common methods, devices, and techniques that may be suggested include short talks or lecturettes, group discussion, reports on related reading or experiences, field trips, projects, panels, sociodramas, dramatic presentation, debates, audiovisual devices such as motion pictures and slides, and tests used for teaching purposes. It is obvious that this list does not represent all of the methods, devices, and techniques that may be called into use to achieve the purpose; however, it is suggestive of the kind of things included in the list. In publishing the unit plan it is not necessary to make a separate list of methods, devices, and techniques for each content item. A single list will avoid duplication.

teaching aids (also see chapter eighteen)

The teaching aids column should list various pieces of equipment, instruments, materials, and essential supplies to be used in carrying out the plans for the methods, devices, and techniques to be used. The list might include such items as projector, screen, film, slides, models, charts—or soap, towel, wash cloth, etc.—as they might be needed in a particular presentation. It would not be necessary, though sometimes desirable, to list specific references such as films by title in this column. Such references should be listed in the appropriate column.

The purpose of this column is to provide a quick inventory of the supplies and equipment needed for any particular method, device, or technique to be used during the course of that phase of the unit. This is important so that the materials can be prepared and tested well ahead of the time they are to be used.

evaluation procedures (also see chapter twenty)

At least two broad classes of evaluation are needed in the evaluation process. First, there is an evaluation of the curriculum and the curriculum process. This will be discussed later. Second, the success of the instruction in achieving the desired expected outcomes must be determined. This evaluation may also contribute to the evaluation of the curriculum. In either case there should be both a quantitative and a qualitative evaluation.

Some kind of measurement and evaluation is necessary to evaluate the teaching. The means of measuring all that should be taught may not always be available; however, the more justifiable criticism is that teachers do not make use of the measuring instruments available and thus their evaluations may not be valid. Furthermore, too often measurement is not associated with evaluation in its broad sense. It is a common experience of students that evaluation comes to be almost synonymous with marking or grading.

The evaluation procedures column, as shown in Figure 8, suggests various means, instruments, devices, and approaches to be used in evaluating the results of instruction in terms of realizing the expected outcomes of specific practices, attitudes, and/or knowledges.

Some of the evaluation procedures that may be included are health knowledge tests, health attitude scales, health practice inventories, personality rating scales, teacher observation, pupil checklists, parent observation, parent checklists, oral and written reports, corrections of remediable deviations or defects, health records, and records of illnesses.

On first thought the reader may want to challenge the use of records of illnesses as a basis of evaluation, particularly if such an evaluation is to form the partial basis for school marks. However, if the goal of health education as stated by the American Association of School Administrators (2:59) is accepted, then the results of such self-direction, or lack of it, can be determined in part by the nature and frequency of some illnesses. For example, success in teaching for immunization can be evaluated, in part, by the fact children do not contract those diseases for which they have been immunized. Of course allowance must be made for the child's dependency on the parents for such immunizations.

references

This column should contain a list of pupil references (by title with essential documentation) including the various books, pamphlets, magazines, films, film strips, slides, and other references that may be called upon in making the learning situation as favorable as possible. Of course the teacher should make certain that they are available to the students. A list of resources of special significance to the teacher should also be suggested under the heading of teacher references. The list of references should be revised regularly, making it possible to keep abreast of the most appropriate, though not always the latest, materials available.

introducing the unit

To enhance the use of the unit the users must be provided with information that will be of assistance to them. This can be done through an introduction that will accompany the unit. Since it will need to reflect the thinking that has gone into the development of the unit, the introduction may well be the last phase of the unit to be completed. However, it should precede the unit in the published document.

The introduction to the unit need not be as extensive as the introduction to the course of study. It contains information that indicates the long range goal of the health problem area, how the unit contributes to attaining that goal, identification of the target group, the length of duration of the unit, a statement of some of the philosophy underlying the unit, including the importance attached to the unit, and any other suggestions that the planners think may be helpful to the teachers who use the plan.

Lesson Planning

Several good approaches have been suggested for developing the lesson plan. If a satisfactory one is in use there may be no reason to change. If the student or teacher is not satisfied with what has been suggested or is interested in a plan that is consistent with the suggested unit plan, then the following plan may be of interest.

The unit plan that has been described can readily be modified into a lesson plan. The resulting lesson plan would consist of the following: (1) a statement of the desired outcome(s) for the lesson, (2) a listing of the content items or subject

139

matter to be used in an attempt to attain the stated outcome(s). This may be a simple topical listing or a more detailed explanation as desired by the teacher. (3) A listing of the methods, devices, and techniques to be used for *each* content item. More than one method should be suggested to provide variety and safeguard against the failure of any method. (4) For each method there should be a list of the teaching aids that will be needed such as a film and projector for an audiovisual presentation. (5) A list of the simple evaluation procedure(s) to be used as the situation warrants. It may not be desirable to try to evaluate results every day. This list should include procedures to be used outside of class as well as those to be used in class. (6) A list of the assignment(s) for the next lesson or lessons.

The lesson plan will differ from the unit plan in the number of expected outcomes to be developed in any one lesson, and there will be a more detailed listing of the subject matter or content to be used in attempting to attain the stated outcome(s). Of course the entire plan is focused on the expected outcome(s) to be stressed in that lesson.

Summary

There is a recognized need for improving the quality of health instruction and considerable agreement that the use of well-planned units of instruction would materially assist in bringing about such improvement. It is recognized that there is no single plan for developing units, but the procedure suggested here has been found to be effective. The seven major divisions suggested are: name or title; outcomes expected in the learner; content; methods, devices, and techniques; teaching aids; evaluation procedures; and references.

In the teaching or instruction unit it is important that emphasis be placed on mastery of a few outcomes rather than on exposure to many. The unit of instruction in health education shoud be planned to emphasize desirable educational outcomes in the areas of *practices, attitudes,* and *knowledge* in keeping with the established criteria of need, interest, comprehension ability, ability to do for one's self, and community values.

References

1. Alberty, Harold, *Reorganizing the High School Curriculum,* Macmillan, New York, 1953.
2. American Association of School Administrators, *Health in Schools, Twentieth Yearbook,* National Education Association, Washington, D.C., 1942.

3. Cauffman, J.G., "Effectiveness of Selected Approaches for the Teaching of Health Education," in Veenker, C.H., Editor, *Synthesis of Research in Selected Areas of Health Instruction,* School Health Education Study, Washington, D.C., 1966.
4. Grout, R.E., *Health Teaching in Schools,* Fifth Edition, Saunders, Philadelphia, 1968.
5. Hopkins, L.T., *Curriculum Principles and Practices,* Sanborn, Chicago, 1934.
6. Johns, E.B., "Guidelines for Health Education Units," *The Journal of the American Association for Health, Physical Education, and Recreation,* 22:6 (1951).
7. Mager, R.F., *Preparing Instructional Objectives,* Fearon, Palo Alto, 1962.
8. Oberteuffer, D., O.A. Harrelson, and M.B. Pollock, *School Health Education,* Harper, New York, 1972.
9. Patty, W.W., *A Health Education Curriculum Summary,* Indiana University Bookstore, Bloomington, out of print.
10. Read D.A. and W.H. Greene, *Creative Teaching in Health,* Second Edition, Macmillan, N.Y., 1975.
11. School Health Education Study, *Health Education, A Conceptual Approach to Curriculum Design,* 3M Press, St. Paul, Minnesota, 1967.
12. Smith, B.O., W.O. Stanley, and J.H. Shores, *Fundamentals of Curriculum Development,* Revised Edition, World, Yonkers-on-Hudson, 1957.
13. Tyler, R.W., *Basic Principles of Curriculum and Instruction,* University of Chicago, Chicago, 1974, c1949.
14. Wood, T.D. and M.O. Lerrigo, *Health Behavior,* Public School, Bloomington, Illinois, 1928.

141

Chapter Thirteen
Expected Outcomes

In spite of the efforts of educators in teacher education programs, in spite of the emphasis on planning that we find in current literature, and in spite of efforts of supervisors and administrators, it is not uncommon to hear the remarks by students, "Why do I have to take health education?" or "We have had that ever since we have been in school." Parents have also expressed a concern that health education courses are not more attractive and beneficial to their children.

If, as we believe, health education is vital and can be one of the most challenging and enlightening experiences in the school life of the child, we must find a way to make it so. It is our contention that proper planning will go a long way toward ensuring the success of the program of health instruction.

As discussed elsewhere, if a curriculum development project is to be successful, proper planning must take place at all three levels of curriculum development. There must be proper planning of the overall school curriculum, including the proper relationship between the different disciplines and other aspects of the school program. There must be proper planning of the curriculum within the disciplines. And there must be proper planning at the course or instructional level, the course of study.

As we are all painfully aware, proper planning at the instructional level implies a great many things, but the first and basic consideration in planning the course of study must be the outcomes hoped for, often called goals or objectives. Since the selection of the expected outcomes sets the pattern for the instruction that is to follow, this selection must be done in the most effective manner possible.

Nature of Expected Outcomes*

The term *expected outcomes* is preferred to the term *objectives* because the former helps focus the entire program on the child. The two terms may be con-

* Also see pages 134–135.

sidered to be synonymous when the term *objective* refers to what happens to and in the child, but in the interest of specificity we have chosen to use the term *expected outcomes*. It is hoped that the common classification of teacher objectives and pupil objectives disappears with the use of the term *expected outcomes*, since they can only be realized by gains in knowledge, changes or reinforcement of attitudes, and changes or reinforcement of behavior on the part of the child. This will enable the goal of health education, intelligent self-direction of health behavior, to be realized.

In considering desirable expected outcomes in health education, it is important to recognize that two levels of learning may be required. These levels may be determined by the nature of the outcomes, and they may also be influenced by the competencies of the learners. For purposes of identification these two levels of learning may be termed *operational* and *analytical*.

Operational learning indicates the fairly simple, routine practices and attitudes that govern day-to-day behavior such as covering the mouth when coughing, brushing teeth, and washing hands. These operational tasks are important to all, and they may comprise the bulk of the learning at lower grade levels and for children of limited capacities.

Analytical learning indicates the deeper understanding of reasons and principles behind the learning. For example, an understanding of certain aspects of physiology, such as phagocytosis, may add meaning and strengthen the learning of an individual. Furthermore, at some later date it may provide the basis for the application of knowledge to the solution of new health problems. Analytical learning will be emphasized as the child matures and for children with the capacity for independent study, research, or simply attainment of the deeper understanding that challenges and adds meaning for the inquiring mind.

Operational learning will generally be manifested by all students at the functional, or doing, level. However, analytical learning may operate at increasingly complex levels including: (1) self-direction, (2) responsibility for the welfare of others, such as child care and home nursing, (3) advisory responsibilities such as health counseling or health instruction, and (4) professional health services such as medicine or nursing. The scope and depth of learning will correspond to the kind and amount of knowledge needed at each level. In any event, however, there is serious need for emphasis on operational learning for all levels, with allowances for the variation that must exist within a level.

Since educational outcomes have commonly been classified into the areas of knowledge, attitudes, and practices (habits or skills), let us examine these to determine their relative contribution to the process of attaining the goal of health education.

Since the goal of health education is expressed as behavior and since behavior in its broad since (including habits of thinking as well as of acting) is influenced by attitudes and knowledges, it follows that the primary concern of health education is to influence behavior. The problem, then, becomes one of selecting the most effective procedures and subject matter in light of the accepted criteria of need, interest, comprehension ability, and dependency with due consideration for community values. In some situations, particularly at the lower grade levels, it will mean placing major emphasis on health practices with less direct emphasis on attitudes and little if any emphasis on basic scientific knowledge concepts. At some times the emphasis may be on attitudes while at other times, particularly in the late high school and/or the college years, the emphasis may be on knowledge. In each instance the real goal is behavior change or reinforcement that will result in healthful living (intelligent self-direction).

Special mention should be made of the role of knowledge in developing expected outcomes. As mentioned elsewhere, knowledge is probably the starting point in developing outcomes at any level. At the preschool and K-1 levels, the knowledge would be very simple, even as simple as "this is what we want you to do." At higher levels reasoning and judgment come into play and the knowledge is at a more complex level such as "diseases may be caused by germs which may get into the food you eat." Starting with basic knowledge, probably as the first expected outcome, the learner is then introduced to attitude and practice outcomes. Here again, they are in harmony with the developmental level of the students. However, the progression is not always from knowledge to attitude to practice. In many instances practices are established, habituated in childhood long before the scientific knowledge could be meaningful. As they are continued the scientific justification for the practices may be learned and the behavior pattern thus strengthened. Cultural dietary patterns serve as a good example of this. Thus a person may eat a healthful diet and feel that the choice is made on the basis of rational judgment when, in fact, the pattern had been well established long before the reasons were understood. It is important to be aware of the impact of pleasant and/or unpleasant experiences on the continuation of the desired practice.

The shifting of emphasis from practices to attitudes to knowledges from grade to grade is a gradual and variable process. No two situations would present the same picture in this respect. A crude picture of the shift and possible relative direct emphasis may be achieved by plotting the respective relative emphases from year to year, as shown in Figure 9.

As the child progresses from grade to grade, there will be a gradual shift from the direct emphasis on practice outcomes in the lower grades to an increasing effort to influence behavior through knowledge at the higher levels. The proportions suggested in this chart should not be taken too literally since they will vary from time to time and place to place.

Perhaps the meaning of some terms should be further clarified. The term *knowledge* is used to mean to be aware of, know, or understand certain items of health information or meaningful expression of facts concerning health. The term *attitude* is used to mean one's feelings, for example what one likes, dislikes,

145

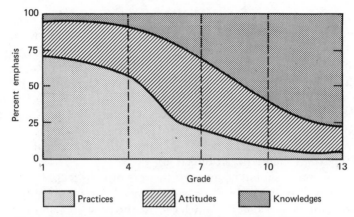

Figure 9. Chart of Changing Emphasis on Expected Outcomes

and enjoys. The term *practice* refers to what one does, the pattern of behavior. In many cases practices may become habits, but the term *practice* is preferred since many of the desirable health behaviors are not readily reduced to the pattern of habitual reaction or habits. To illustrate this with an example we need only cite the desirable practice of seeing one's dentist twice a year. Such behavior could hardly be said to become a habit since it is not done without conscious thought and planning.

The very close relationship of attitudes and behavior should not be overlooked. However, it should not be assumed that all health behavior is synonymous with the corresponding health attitude, since certain health behavior may stem from attitudes that are not health related attitudes at all. For example, the teenager who brushes his teeth after eating may do so, not because of his attitude toward dental health, but because he wants to make a favorable impression on his girl friend.

Likewise, teenage health behavior in relation to the use of certain habit-forming substances commonly stems from social motivation rather than the motivation of health attitudes. For example, the motivation for experimenting with drugs is often peer pressure.

If knowledge and attitude outcomes are expected to promote desirable practice outcomes, what should be the nature of the expected outcomes in these areas? Desirable knowledge outcomes should be those classes of information that are directly related to or are necessary for the establishment of the desirable practices in related areas, as was so ably pointed out by Wood and Lerrigo. (16:25) The knowledge items should have a close relationship to the actual practice. Furthermore, it follows that the complexity or level of the knowledge will vary from grade to grade, but some knowledge is basic to the development of attitudes. Attitude outcomes should be reflected in healthful behavior. They should be selected on that basis.

146

Perhaps a word about the function of stated expected outcomes is in order. It is sometimes suggested that they serve as a guide to selection of content and methods, devices, and techniques. In a sense this is true, but a more accurate assessment would be that the expected outcomes serve as a means of meeting the health education needs and interests of the students. In turn the content and methods, devices, and techniques are selected for their relevance in making this possible.

One of the most important considerations in planning the unit is the number of outcomes to be expected. In planning an instruction unit it is a common temptation to list a great many expected outcomes. It is a much wiser procedure to select a few (indeed, a very few) outcomes to be expected and develop them in many different ways than it is to list a great many outcomes and then to fail to develop any of them satisfactorily.

Ordinarily, the number of expected outcomes will be directly related to the length of the unit. However, it is conceivable that some outcomes, though few in number, might require a considerable amount of time for mastery, resulting in a long unit. This would be especially true for practice outcomes. Also, it is important that there be followup instruction to reinforce units previously taught. It might be correct to assume that a unit may range in length from a few days to as much as six weeks. If shorter than a few days it would be little more than a lesson, while if longer than one-third of a semester it probably should be divided into subtopics that could well be developed as units themselves.

Expressing Expected Outcomes*

Since there are only three kinds of expected educational outcomes, knowledge, attitudes, and practices, it would seem to be a simple matter to express them clearly and succinctly. However, this does not seem to be the common experience of curriculum planners.

No doubt some of the difficulty stems from the fact than in many areas of education the emphasis has been on knowledge outcomes. While this should not be true in health education, it has been common practice to think mainly in terms of knowledge. Such thinking has been supported and encouraged by the difficulty of evaluating the success of attaining attitude and practice outcomes.

If the goals of health education are to be attained, more emphasis must be placed on attitude (affective) and practice (behavioral) outcomes. Oberteuffer et al. suggested that:

> *a properly stated behavioral objective, most authorities agree, satisfies these criteria: (1) It is stated in terms of the learner, not in terms of the teacher's intentions; (2) it is operational, in that the learner can practice the behavior and measurably demonstrate his [sic] new ability or change in belief in the*

* Also see Pages 134–135.

147

classroom; (3) it specifies a single behavior and a single content area. Whether it is broadly stated or narrowly defined depends upon its function in the curriculum plan. (12:60–61)

Mager has stressed the importance of the wording of the objective. One of the important considerations that he stressed was to incorporate the evaluation process in the statement of the objective. In his final summary regarding instructional objectives Mager pointed out the following:

1. A statement of instructional objectives is a collection of words or symbols describing one of your educational intents.
2. An objective will communicate your interest to the degree you have described what the learner will be DOING when demonstrating his a- chievement and how you will know when he is doing it.
3. To describe terminal behavior (what the learner will be DOING):
   a. Identify and name the over-all behavior act.
   b. Define the important conditions under which the behavior is to occur (givens or restrictions, or both).
   c. Define the criteria of acceptable performance.
4. Write a separate statement for each objective; the more statements you have, the better chance you have of making clear your intent.
5. If you give the learner a copy of your objectives you may not have to do much more. (11:53)

The almost insurmountable difficulty of writing an attitude expected out- come is readily apparent when one tries to express the expected attitude behavior to include the evaluative criteria. In expressing attitude outcomes there is the temptation to use a statement such as "the student has a wholesome attitude toward health." It is readily apparent that this statement does not give a criterion for a *wholesome* attitude. A more satisfactory statement would be "the student wants to be healthy" or "the student wants to avoid contracting a (specific) com- municable disease." However, this statement does not give the criteria for accep- table performance but it does reflect the desired specific behavior. The criteria for acceptable performance will be discovered by the student as the content is developed. Furthermore, since the expected outcomes are being prepared for a real live teacher, not a teaching machine, (10) there is opportunity for explanation and interpretation by the teacher. In the unit plan that we propose, we do not at- tempt to limit the statements of expected outcomes to a particular form or pattern as long as they comply with the criteria suggested by Oberteuffer. (12:60–61) Evaluation of attitude outcomes will be discussed later. In the meantime it is im- portant to recognize the importance of attitudes in their relation to health behavior. The difficulty of evaluating them does not negate the importance of working to that end. It would be easier to express attitudes in terms of long range goals and thus avoid the necessity for immediate evaluation. However, long range goals can be attained only through the route of immediate objectives.

The same difficulty is not experienced in the knowledge and practice realms. This fact probably accounts for the tendency to emphasize knowledge and practice outcomes, whereas the attitude is undoubtedly the most important concern in influencing behavior.

Curriculum developers may well consider Mager's recommendations for expressing expected outcomes (objectives) and apply them whenever practical. The difficulty encountered in expressing attitude outcomes and in dealing with the evaluation of attitudes should in no way discourage attitudes from being considered as expected outcomes. Other methods of evaluation can be used.

Knowledge and practice expected outcomes are simple and are easily expressed. In the case of knowledge, the expressions *knows* or *understands* are commonly used. If Mager's recommendations are followed the statements will include the criteria of acceptable performance. For example, an expected knowledge outcome in nutrition might be, *can list five classes of foods.*

Expected practice outcomes may be expressed in the simple statement of what practice is expected. For example, desirable personal cleanliness outcomes might be expressed as *washes hands after going to the toilet, brushes or rinses teeth after eating,* or *covers the mouth and nose with tissue when sneezing.*

Expected attitude outcomes can be expressed through the use of such terms as enjoys, likes, dislikes, and wants. For example, a desirable personal cleanliness attitude outcome might be expressed as *enjoys being neat and clean.* The Mager approach might be used through a statement such as: "given the opportunity, the student elects to wear clean clothes." While this is actually a practice it does reflect an attitude.

Whenever an expected outcome is expressed, the learner should be able to clearly perceive the behavior that is expected, whether that behavior be knowledge, attitude, or practice. However, there may be times when it is not desirable for the learner to be aware of the expected outcome. In cases where an undesirable attitude needs to be changed, more may be accomplished by quietly fostering an environment conducive to the desired attitude and by reinforcing desirable behaviors than by a confrontation that may more firmly establish the undesirable behavior. This is especially true of young children.

In recent years there has been considerable emphasis on Bloom's Taxonomy of Educational Objectives, both in the cognitive and affective domains. According to Krathwohl et al. (9:186–193) the two divisions of the cognitive domain are knowledge and intellectual abilities. They classify knowledge as knowledge: of specific facts, of ways and means of dealing with specifics, and of the universals and abstractions in a field. The intellectual abilities include comprehension, application, analysis, synthesis, and evaluation.

In the affective domain Krathwohl et al. (9:63–67, 176–185) describe five levels: receiving, responding, valuing, organization, and characterization by a value or value complex. There are sublevels within each of these levels, which we will indicate in the following example of how to approach the use of a taxonomy of educational objectives in the area of nutrition.

taxonomy of educational objectives regarding the relationship between nutrition and health

1.0 Receiving
    1.1 Is conscious of a possible relationship between diet and health: *Awareness.*
    1.2 Is tolerant of a variety of foods: *Willingness to receive.*
    1.3 Is alert for the presence of a variety of foods that may have an impact on health: *Controlled or selected attention.*

2.0 Responding
    2.1 Complies with requests to eat a variety of foods: *Acquiescence in responding.*
    2.2 Voluntarily looks for variety in foods served: *Willingness to respond.*
    2.3 Enjoys eating a variety of foods: *Satisfaction in response.*

3.0 Valuing
    3.1 Believes that what one eats affects one's health: *Acceptance of a value.*
    3.2 Voluntarily looks for foods that provide variety in the diet: *Preference for a value.*
    3.3 Seeks out, or selects, and eats a varied diet: *Commitment.*

4.0 Organization
    4.1 Attempts to identify the characteristics of a healthful diet: *Conceptualization of a value.*
    4.2 Develops a plan for regulating one's diet in accordance with the body needs: *Organization of a value system.*

5.0 Characterization by a Value or Value Complex
    5.1 Views health problems according to their possible relation to diet: *Generalized set.*
    5.2 Develops a value system consistent with what is known about the relationship of diet and health: *Characterization.*

The progression from being conscious of a relationship between diet and health to developing a value system indicates the kind of progression that is necessary in developing a concept. In order to achieve that end subconcepts, long range goals, and behavioral objectives will need to be developed, and the progress will not always follow the exact pattern suggested in the above example. However, recognition of the need for progression is important and should be taken into consideration in unit planning.

Criteria for Selecting Expected Outcomes*

The suggestion that the knowledge will vary from grade to grade implies the need for considering the criteria for selecting the expected outcomes and the problem areas to be considered in the health instructional program. As stated elsewhere, the criteria proposed are *need, interest, comprehension ability, dependency* (ability to act independently), and *community values*. The first three of these are commonly suggested as criteria. However, it seems that any program designed to bring about changes in behavior or reinforce desirable behavior must,also consider the possibility of putting into practice the desired behavior. Using the criterion of *dependency,* if other factors are equal, it is logical to emphasize the desired outcomes that the learner can do something about independently, as a result of individual efforts, without depending on someone else.

The criterion of *community values* has its base in the mores of the community. It operates most commonly in the controversial areas. In such areas little good can be accomplished in the face of strong opposition or rejection by the community. This criterion suggests that there may be some health problem areas you would like to include in your teaching but that the community is not prepared to accept.

To illustrate how to use the criteria in planning the health education program, let us look at the *needs* of children just entering school. It should be obvious that their health education needs will be directly related to their developmental level and the tasks they will need to perform in the development process, the developmental tasks. Furthermore, as pointed out by Gagné (6:168–174), there are two aspects to the criterion of need that must be considered: What prerequisites to the desired learning are already mastered and what prerequisites are still needed? This strongly supports the need for competent diagnostic testing or evaluation to determine the needs of each student. Gagne also indicated that once something has been learned, periodic and spaced reviews are more important than repetition, a practice in strengthening that learning. One of the major tasks of the child entering school is to achieve a new level of independence. This is achieved by realizing some essential minor accomplishments, one of which is the need to get to and from school safely. This need (the criterion of *need)* strongly suggests that the safety of the child pedestrian in going to and from school should be a major consideration very early in the school life of the child. Hence, a unit of

* Also see page 134–135.

151

health and safety instruction may be planned, and taught, that will attempt to develop intelligent self-direction of health and safety behavior, for example, when a pedestrian, when boarding buses, or when getting into and out of cars.

The criterion of *need,* which is the primary guide, must be viewed according to the characteristics of the students. As the characteristics vary from individual to individual, grade to grade, and community to community the needs will vary. It follows, then, that the first step in planning the health education curriculum is to get a clear understanding of the characteristics of the students. This should include an assessment of their previous educational experiences through such procedures as diagnostic tests, the study of previous anecdotal records, and student evaluation of needs as related to their experiences.

The use of the criterion of *interest* may be illustrated in reference to the developmental task of achieving satisfactory social relationships. The interest of adolescents in the opposite sex provides the basis for planning units of instruction that can assist students in accomplishing this developmental task. Of course the wise teacher will not limit instruction to the interests of students. The needs associated with those interests will also be considered. Furthermore, if the need is present the effective teacher can do much to motivate interest.

The criterion of *comprehension ability* suggests that the subject matter must be understandable and understood by the students. It is readily apparent that vocabulary, ideas, and level of understanding must be commensurate with the intellectual development of the student. This criterion deals more with the nature and detail of subject matter than with the actual problem. People of all ages have problems of social adjustment, but the problem is expressed and dealt with on a level indicated by the comprehension ability of the individual. For example in the lower grades the problem of being accepted may be solved by including the child in group activities while in adolescence acceptance may involve such relationships as age, sex, academic achievement, and social standing, resulting in a much more complex problem that requires the cooperation of various school personnel such as counselors, administrators, other teachers, and other students.

The criterion of *dependency* is closely related to maturity level of the individual. As mentioned earlier this criterion suggests that the major emphasis should be placed on expected outcomes for which the child can be independent. This may suggest that since a child must depend on the parents the wise teacher puts less emphasis than would otherwise be desired on a particular practice when it is known that the parents may not cooperate. The criterion of dependency suggests that the emphasis be placed on things the child can do without having to depend on someone else. For example, let us consider the wisdom of laying great stress on the particular practice of visiting the dentist twice each year when, as the result of limited finances, there is no opportunity to follow the desired practice, as is true in many homes. Perhaps it should be pointed out that the criterion of dependency does not suggest that the desirability of a practice or practices not be taught. It does suggest that great importance be attached to desired outcomes for which the learner can be independent, while those desirable outcomes which are not feasible at that particular time be postponed until they are feasible or that they be emphasized from the point of view of desirability when possible.

The criterion of *community values* can be used to guide the teacher along lines permissible, if not wholly acceptable, in the community. It does not suggest avoiding controversial areas; it only suggests a careful approach. Seldom, if ever, would all aspects of a controversial subject be rejected by a community. The clue to successful introduction of important aspects of a controversial area rests with the ability of the planners to identify these acceptable aspects and to include them in the program. At the same time the community may be brought to see the importance of and to accept other important health considerations that they may have been rejecting. The effective approach is to feel one's way in controversial areas, bringing the community along as rapidly as it is able to move. Community participation in planning is essential in such areas.

It is important for the health educator to realize that all desirable health practices will not be developed in one generation. This point is illustrated by the seemingly hopeless experience of an elementary school teacher who felt that she had failed in attempting to teach practices of cleanliness and neatness, only to find a few years later that the children of her "failures" were neat and clean.

The criterion of *need* doubtless takes precedence if an order of importance of the criteria is to be suggested. It is true that comprehension ability and interest are both important, but the competent health education teacher can certainly adjust the level of the subject matter to the comprehension ability of the student and/or stimulate interest when it is not evident. Furthermore, it does not seem to be out of order to assume that the health education teacher who is concerned with the welfare of students will go to considerable effort to do something about dependency when the other criteria are present. For example, the teacher should be aware of possible sources of assistance in securing needed corrections of defects, such as glasses, while the ingenious teacher may work out a plan for regular use of physical education shower facilities for interested students lacking these facilities in their own homes. In similar manner, the teacher who is concerned with the need for instruction in controversial areas will not give up in the face of community attitudes that preclude certain instructional areas. Such a teacher will seek ways of approaching the problem to provide possibilities for such instruction, even on a limited basis, while at the same time working to open minds to the importance of such instruction. For example, a study of sex education may be approached through discussions in the health committee of the P.T.S.A., possibly leading to a study of community needs in this problem area.

Since the relative importance of the criteria used in selecting the expected outcomes will be influenced by the characteristics of the children, it becomes important to recognize those characteristics. It follows that the first step in planning a unit for any group of children is to understand the characteristics of the children. When the characteristics of the children are identified, it is then possible to identify their health needs. And when the health needs are known the health education needs can be identified. It is then possible, and only then, to move on to selecting the desired expected outcomes that form the basis of all unit planning, either for instructional units or for resource units.

As indicated in Chapter 12, additional procedures to be used in selecting expected outcomes might be analysis of needs of the children; pupil expressions of interest; observation of pupil interests; opinions of other health educators, health service staff, and parents; study of the practices as revealed in other courses of study; study of research findings; and practicality.

Joint Planning for Health Education

Pupil participation in planning for health education should be encouraged. It is safe to assume that the greatest contribution pupil participation in planning makes is the arousing of interests or motivation of the students. It would be absurd to suppose that the well-prepared teacher would not soon know what problem areas to include in the study. However, it is almost equally absurd to leave the wishes of students out of consideration. The wise teacher will participate in pupil planning, thus making it "our course."

The participation of parents in the planning procedure is commonly neglected. Too often teachers are inclined to feel that parents do not want to have a part in planning or, at the other extreme, they may fear that parents may want to dictate what is taught. The actual facts of the case are, undoubtedly, somewhere in between these two extremes. Febel (5) found that parents whom he interviewed were generally in agreement with the efforts being made by the school in the area of health education and, furthermore, there was a marked interest in those efforts and a desire on the part of many to discuss the problems. Charlson (2) found that senior students, parents, and clergy all favored providing sex education in the schools. These studies serve to illustrate the value of communication with parents, and others, both in planning the curriculum and in supporting an ongoing program. It is one important means of determining whether the schools are meeting the needs of the community. Furthermore, if there is resistance among parents to what is being taught, school teachers and administrators should know it.

Teachers should realize that most parents are genuinely interested in the welfare of their children and that the areas of question or disagreement generally have to do with minor points. The teacher will be in a much better position to conduct an educational program, including adult education, if the wishes of the parents (including the taboos) are known. Furthermore, the chances of the success of home-school cooperation, which is so essential in health education, will be very much enhanced if the parents have had a part, even though a minor one, in making the plans.

The medical profession and related professional groups should also take part in making the broad plans for any program so vitally concerned with health. This can probably best be carried out at the policymaking level, that is, through the health council and/or committee, but it is important that the teacher have reliable sources to call on for certain kinds of information. In a field that is changing as rapidly as the health field, it is difficult to keep up with new developments. Consequently, the cooperation of those in the health sciences is vital to the continued effective functioning of the health education program.

Teaching for Health Through Ability Achievement

In considering the problem of ability achievement as contrasted with ability grouping, it is important to remember that *achievement* is the product of many factors. Some of these are intelligence, aptitude, interest, effort, and opportunity. *Ability* is also a product of several factors including intelligence, aptitude, and opportunity with the result that there are many kinds of abilities. This fact complicates the grouping of students by ability because we must ask the question: what ability?

In an attempt to provide for achievement in harmony with ability, the concept of ability achievement or achievement independence is being suggested. In a given time achievement will vary, and may be caused to vary, according to the factors that influence achievement. Provision must be made for wide variation of achievement within the typical classroom of America. The advantages of grouping for health instruction are recognized. The question is simply: what kind of grouping? Although homogeneous ability grouping has been in common use for a long time [St. Louis, 1867 (15)] and in spite of overwhelming support of the practice, Wilson and Schmits (15:535–536) reported that the research does not support the assumption that ability grouping aids achievement. They pointed out that it may in fact be damaging to the social and emotional growth (health) of children. Therefore, what can be done to make possible the successful instruction in healthful living in groups (classes) of widely varying abilities?

Instead of grouping students on the basis of homogeneous ability groups, the use of small heterogeneous ability groups will allow for optimum individual achievement while at the same time minimizing the possible negative effects of the labeling that inevitably accompanies ability grouping. Within the heterogeneous groups we can think of three gradations of achievement: *minimum, general,* and *special.*

Minimum achievement should be expected of all members of the health class. Certain members will not achieve beyond this level. Having expended an optimum amount of energy at maximum concentration for the specified period of time, people with less than average natural endowment (I.Q. of 70–90) will have reached their maximum achievement. This will generally not measure up to the achievement of those with the greater natural endowment. For example, the minimum achievement student may never be able to plan and prepare meals, select health services, etc. However, their achievement should fall short in quantity rather than in quality. What they learn they should learn well. Desirable health practices should be well established.

General achievement should be expected of all those in the higher achievement level classification. For the greater proportion of the students at this level (I.Q. 90–110) this will be their maximum achievement. Again, what is learned should be learned well. Those students should master what is learned at both the minimum and the general achievement levels. The learning at the minimum level will be comparable to the learning of the minimum achievement group. However, the general achievement group should go well beyond the minimum achievement group in quantity of learning.

Special achievement should be expected of the gifted or superior student (I.Q. above 110). This should include all achievement at the minimum and general levels, but it should go beyond them in quantity and complexity.

The increase in quantity of achievement from level to level might be characterized as an expanding achievement. Each successively higher level of ability should go higher and deeper in achievement. Some indication of the differences in the levels may be gathered from Figure 10.

Each successive level of achievement in Figure 10 incorporates the achievements of the previous levels. Graphically, this progression might be represented as shown in Figure 11.

Identification of the expected outcomes at each level remains the crucial problem for course of study committees.

Meaningful health instruction in this heterogeneous class situation must provide for challenging learning situations for all concerned. The successful teacher can organize the class activities to provide for supervision and direction of the learning activities of the dependent students, motivation and development of self-direction of those only partially independent, and guidance for those who are able to work independently (e.g., research projects) either individually or in groups. This calls for a high degree of flexibility within the class. At times homogeneous groupings may be desirable while at other times it may be desirable to have small heterogeneous groupings, particularly if pupil-to-pupil cooperation or assistance is desired.

Levels	Goals	Through

III.
Special
Achievement
	Physiological,
	psychological, and
	sociological
	foundations
		Science fairs
		Research
		Creative
		  writing
		Supplementary
		  reading

II.
General
Achievement
	More complex knowledge,
	attitudes, and practices.
	Simple scientific
	foundations.
		Simple
		  experiments
		Supplementary
		  reading
		Demonstrations
		Projects

I. Minimum Achievement	Simple basic knowledge, attitudes, and practices	Practical daily application

Figure 10. Levels of Achievement by Abilities.

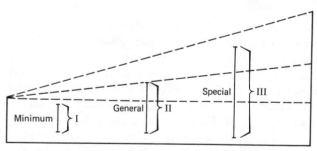

Figure 11. Achievement Expectations by Ability Level.

It should not be necessary to point out that the learning activities at the special achievement level will usually take them far from the beaten path of the textbook, and in many instances far from the classroom. While all health instruction should be in harmony with the needs and interests of the students as they relate to developmental levels, and to developmental tasks for those levels, it is especially important that the independent students be guided along lines compatible with the developmental tasks they are facing.

157

The Conceptual Approach in Health Education

Two variations of the traditional "outcome" approach that have been proposed are noted here. Cushman (4) emphasized the importance of *developmental tasks* as the prime consideration in planning for health instruction. This proposal does not preclude the use of the traditional expected outcomes of knowledge, attitudes, and practices. It emphasizes the significance of the relationship of selected expected outcomes to the developmental tasks facing the learner.

The second variation of the traditional approach is the emphasis on the *conceptual approach*. This approach was used by the Curriculum Commission of the Division of Health Education of the American Association for Health, Physical Education, and Recreation in developing guidelines for health education.(8) The conceptual approach was further developed into a conceptual model by the writing team of the School Health Education Study for the Curriculum Development Project under the direction of Elena M. Sliepcevich. (13)

The conceptual approach is based on the recognized principle that the perceptions of the individual provide the basis for learning. A concept is defined as a relatively complete and meaningful idea in the mind of the person. It is the subjective product of that person's way of making meaningful things seen or otherwise perceived in experience.

The conceptual model developed in the School Health Education Study (13) suggested six levels of hierarchy. At the first level *health* is the comprehensive, unified concept. At the second level three *key concepts of growing and developing, decision making,* and *interacting* are thought to be the unifying threads of the curriculum that characterize the processes underlying health. Emerging from these key concepts at the third level are 10 concept that are viewed as the major organizing elements of the curriculum or indicators from the direction of the learning experience. At the fourth level 33 subconcepts, categorized under the *concepts,* serve as guides to select and order the substance of health education. At the fifth level or order of the hierarchy come the *goals* related to each of the 10 concepts and viewed in the three domains of behavior: cognitive (knowledge), affective (attitudes), and action (practices). *Behavioral outcomes* are shown at the bottom of the hierarchy. These are developed in the more detailed instructional materials, in appropriate relationship to the four levels of progression, rather than by grade levels. These four levels correspond to the four major grade level divisions of our schools.

The conceptual framework for health education is characterized by: adaptability to different grade levels; flexibility to allow for individual differences and differences in community needs; and permanence that provides a framework to allow for the discovery of new knowledge and its inclusion in the health education curriculum within the suggested framework.

158

In view of what seems to be a general movement toward the use of concepts in curriculum writing it should be pointed out that there is no conflict between the approach we are suggesting and the concept approach. As demonstrated in the School Health Education Study, if the concept approach is used there is still need for planning at the expected outcome (behavioral objectives) level. (13:95-192) Behavioral objectives contribute to attaining long range goals. The concepts and subconcepts provide the framework within which the teaching-learning process takes place whereas the long range goals and behavioral objectives represent the desired behaviors.

The relationship of the various levels in the conceptual approach may be seen by examining one of the concepts. For example, for the concept "food selection and eating patterns are determined by physical, social, mental, economic, and cultural factors," three subconcepts are listed: (1) Choice of foods determines nutritional balance; (2) a balanced diet affects well being and the desire for the well being affects food choices, and (3) food selection and eating patterns serve social and psychological purposes as well as filling physiological needs. For each of these subconcepts content is suggested for each of the three dimensions: physical, mental, and social.

In this manner the framework is established within which the planners move on into the long range goals and behavioral outcomes. These are listed by progression level with references to the appropriate subconcepts for each behavioral objective. Each level embodies an increasing complex level of attainment. Also for each level a sequence of behavioral objectives is suggested, making for progression within the level. (13:90-93) The unit plan we are suggesting would be applicable at the long range goal and behavioral outcome level, and it is applicable within the conceptual framework.

As was pointed out in *Health Education* (13:xiv) the conceptual approach is one suggested approach to curriculum development. There may be other approaches that are more satisfactory for the individuals involved. For some it may be more meaningful to think of *principles of health*, rather than health concepts. For example a nutrition principle might be expressed as "health depends, in part, on the food you eat." This principle might be developed in the same line as a concept.

The conceptual framework, as developed in the School Health Education Study, should be helpful in promoting the effectiveness and status of health education by furnishing a uniform approach to health education within a framework that allows for the differences essential to success in modifying behavior. Instructional materials that have been designed for use in the conceptual approach may be secured from the 3M Educational Press. (13)

Importance of The Teacher

The teacher is the most important single factor in the classroom. The successful teacher is motivated by a sincere desire to be of service. The teacher will bring to the classroom an abundance of common sense, a genuine interest in the welfare of mankind, an understanding of the other person's point of view, a respect for the right of the other person to hold that point of view, a concern for discovering new truths and better ways of doing things, and a sound preparation in the basic health sciences coupled with a deep understanding of human behavior and mastery of educational method.

Procedures for joint planning such as discussions, the question box, surveys, diagnostic knowledge and attitude tests, and health examination reports are all valuable. However, the final responsibility for the success of the educational experience rests squarely on the shoulders of the teacher.

Content in Relation to Expected Outcomes

Although the outcomes that are realized are the most important consideration in health instruction, those outcomes have a direct relationship to the content used in attaining them. To a considerable degree, the outcomes are dependent on the content. In many instances the expected outcomes are vague ideas in the minds of the learners, if they are aware of them at all. The content is in more concrete form and it provides the learner with specific material that is capable of being manipulated, tried, and understood.

what is content?

In the unit plan the content is the subject matter that is used. It is *what is studied* in the process of reaching the goal, the expected outcome. As has been pointed out, at times it may be desirable to hide the expected outcome from the learner, particularly if it involves giving up some habit to establish another; but content is never hidden. It is the nourishment provided for the purpose of nurturing the development of the desired outcome. As previously indicated, the nature of the content depends on several factors such as nature of the expected outcome, the specificity of the expected outcome, and the developmental level of the learner.

In reference to the nature of the expected outcomes, content intended to foster the development of knowledge may consist of simple factual information while content intended to foster the development of attitudes and practices will often need to have emotional connotations, stimulating the identification of the learner with the desired attitude to the extent that the attitude becomes a force strong enough to influence behavior.

In reference to the specificity of the expected outcome, content intended to foster the development of a simple outcome, such as brushing the teeth after eating or understanding what makes teeth decay, may be simple and factual and need not be complex. However, if the expected outcome is complex in nature, such as selecting or preparing and eating wholesome meals, the content will need to be broad in scope and more detailed in facts. Furthermore, since the outcome involves practices the content must include value connotations that may have emotional implications that will serve to provide goals toward which the individual may progress.

In reference to the developmental level of the learner, it is obvious that content must be within the comprehension ability of the learner. This criterion relates to how the content is presented and to what is presented. In the area of dental health it is important that the learner understand the desirability of clean teeth, but the depth of understanding varies from a simple realization that it is desirable to a fuller understanding of the nature of the process of tooth decay and the factors that contribute to decay. In the higher grades this may involve simple chemistry, physiology of digestion, and an understanding of tooth structure.

how is content indicated?

In the unit plan the suggested content may be listed in a number of ways ranging from a simple topical listing of content areas to a somewhat lengthy description of factual information. The form of presentation must depend in part on the people for whom the unit is being prepared and the knowledge possessed by the teachers. If the unit is being prepared for use by teachers who are well prepared in the subject, a simple topical listing of content areas will suffice. As the knowledge of the teacher decreases the detail of content must be increased. For the teacher whose preparation in the field is limited it will be necessary to provide enough detail of content to give direction to the instruction. This need not duplicate the content of the resource materials (e.g., references and textbooks), but it must guide the teacher in the use of such resources. For the well-informed teacher it may be sufficient to use the topical item, causes of tooth decay as the content item, but for the teacher who is not well prepared it will be desirable to add subtopics such as bacteria, plaque, and carbohydrates so that pertinent topics be included. The detail of content needed in the unit plan will depend on the competency of the user. As Oberteuffer et al. pointed out, "the content should expand but not go beyond that prescribed in the objective." (12:113)

how many content items are needed?

Two of the most important principles related to learning are *exercise* (use and disuse) and *effect*. Practical application of these principles to unit planning suggests that development of an expected outcome, especially a practice, will be realized most successfully if there is sufficient desirable exposure to or repetition of the desired learning. This suggests the important principle for unit planning that *there should be several items of content for each expected outcome.* In practical applications this means we should use a variety of approaches both of content and of method to insure the attainment of the desired results.

If the principle of *effect* is to be observed, it will dictate that different items of content be used in instruction that is intended to develop different expected outcomes. Hence, the same items of content would not be repeated even though the expected outcomes were closely related. In instances where this might seem to be desirable the expected outcomes should be reexamined to make certain that there are, in fact, two or more different expected outcomes. If the expected outcomes duplicate each other, one of them should be eliminated. If there are two or more distinct expected outcomes, then the scope of the content should be examined to determine whether it may not be too broad. In most instances it will be found that certain aspects of the content item in question apply more specifically to one expected outcome and other aspects to another. In such cases the scope of the content items may be reduced, using information that is most applicable for each expected outcome.

Use of identical information for more than one expected outcome should be avoided. Although the same basic information may be helpful in developing more than one outcome, such repetition serves to strengthen the common criticism that there is much repetition in our health teaching. Furthermore, the use of a variety of content items promotes habit formation without boring repetition, and it allows for individual differences that make different approaches necessary.

why is content important?

The importance of selecting content that is specifically intended to promote the development of a particular outcome is stressed because of the common practice, and weakness, in planning of thinking only in terms of content (what to teach) rather than in terms of desirable results (expected outcomes). When selection of teaching material (subject matter) is based on the content approach, the possibilities of planning the instruction to meet the needs of a specific learner are seriously limited. Too often the content approach results in amassing a large store of information, much of which has no particular value in the struggle to conserve health. When planning is approached from the point of view of meeting the needs of the learner, in terms of developing desirable outcomes, it is possible to eliminate much information that has no particular value to the learner. Furthermore, the content approach to planning for health instruction is seriously limited in developing desirable attitudes and practices.

Content is important, but unless it supports the realization of the expected outcome it is of little or no value. In selecting content it is helpful to refer to lists of health topics such as those compiled by Byrd (1:89–95) and Hardt (7:656–660). The topics were arranged by categories, and they can be a useful resource for identifying content items that may be used in developing the desired outcomes. Other sources of content items, and of specific content, include research reports in professional journals, public health service and state health department literature, local health department personnel and publications, professional health agencies such as the American Medical Association and the American Dental Association, voluntary agency publications and consultants, foundations and institutes, sponsored agencies, and textbooks.

Since the content provides the basic ideas, and ideals, for fostering the attainment of the expected outcomes, and since such information is essential to the development of the outcomes, it is apparent that content ranks next to expected outcomes in significance in the unit plan. To a very great degree the commonly accepted criteria that apply to selection of expected outcomes also apply to the selection of content. These are *needs, interests, comprehension ability, dependency of the learners,* and *community values.*

Summary

Proper planning at the instructional level is strongly dependent on the selection of the most appropriate expected outcomes or objectives. The expected outcomes of knowledge, attitudes, and practices will differ in nature depending on whether the learning is operational or analytical. Furthermore, the emphasis on the different kinds of outcomes will vary from grade to grade.

While there is a strong trend toward expressing expected outcomes in behavioral terms, this should not preclude the stating of desirable expected outcomes that cannot be readily expressed as overt behavior.

The criteria of need, interest, comprehension ability, dependence, and community values should be supplemented by other procedures that may be helpful in selecting the expected outcomes. Since the typical classroom will contain individuals of a wide range of abilities, there must be some arrangement for individuals to achieve according to their own abilities. This we have called ability achievement.

In specific reference to the items of content, three considerations seem to stand out in importance. (1) Is the content directly related to the expected outcome in such a way as to promote its attainment in the learner. (2) Are there sufficient different items of content for each expected outcome to allow for desirable emphasis without boring repetition and for individual differences among learners. (3) Does the content item and the subject matter suggested by the item meet the accepted criteria? If these three major conditions are met, there is reasonable assurance of a sound basis for instruction intended to conserve health.

References

1. Byrd, O.E., "The Health Curriculum: 500 topics," *The Journal of School Health,* 28:3 (1958).

2. Charlson, V.R., *The Need for Family Life Education on the Secondary School Level,* unpublished doctoral dissertation, Indiana University, 1962.

3. Committee on Health Guidance in Sex Education, *Growth Patterns and Sex Education,* American School Health Association, Kent, Ohio, (1967).

4. Cushman, W.P., "Developmental Tasks—A Source of Health Problems," *The Journal of School Health,* 29:7 (1959).

5. Febel, Frederick, *Parental Opinion Survey of Health education on the Secondary Public School Level,* unpublished doctoral dissertation, Indiana University, 1954.

6. Gagné, R.M., "Some New Views of Learning and Instruction," in Hass, G., *Curriculum Planning: A New Approach,* Allyn & Bacon, Boston, 1977.

7. Hardt, D.V., "Health Curriculum: 370 Topics," *The Journal of School Health,* 48:1 (1978).

8. *Health Concepts,* American Association for Health, Physical Education, and Recreation, Washington, D.C., 1967.

9. Krathwohl, D.R., B.S. Bloom, and B.B. Masia, *Taxonomy of Educational Objectives, The Classification of Educational Goals, Handbook II, Affective Domain,* McKay, N.Y., 1964.

10. Mager, R.F., *Preparing Objectives for Programmed Instruction,* Fearon, San Francisco, 1956.

11. Mager, R.F., *Preparing Instructional Objectives,* Fearon, Palo Alto, California, 1962.

12. Oberteuffer, D., O.A. Harrelson, and M.B. Pollock, *School Health Education,* Harper, New York, 1972.

13. School Health Education Study, *Health Education, A Conceptual Approach to Curriculum Design,* 3M, St. Paul, 1967.

14. Vargas, J.S., *Writing Worthwhile Behavioral Objectives,* Harper & Row, New York, 1972.

15. Wilson, B.J., and D.W. Schmits, "What's New in Ability Grouping?" *Phi Delta Kappan,* 59:8 (1978).

16. Wood, T.D., and M.O. Lerrigo, *Health Behavior,* Public School, Bloomington, Illinois, 1928.

Chapter Fourteen
Health Education Through Healthful School Living and Health Services

As indicated earlier, experiences in the healthful environment and health services are basic components of the health education curriculum. However, without careful planning and supervision those experiences may fail to contribute to healthful living. In fact they may have a negative influence in this regard. In this chapter we will explore some ways by which the environmental and health service experiences may contribute to the goal of health education.

Healthful School Living

Until fairly recently this phase of the school health program was called healthful school living. With the publication of the revision of the National Education Association—American Medical Association book, *Healthful School Environment* (4) in 1969, the use of the term *environment* was accepted in place of the term *living*. In the opinion of the present writers the terms are interchangeable, but since it is more logical to think of a program of healthful living rather than a program of healthful environment, the term *healthful living* is being used in connection with the instructional emphasis in health education. By definition, the health education curriculum includes planned learning experiences in all aspects of the school program, including experiences related to the healthful environment in the school. Experiences in the healthful environment are very commonly identified as *activities* and/or *situations.*

There is some evidence as gained from textbooks, professional journal articles, and other printed materials, that the concept of the fourfold nature of health as physical, emotional, social, and spiritual well-being is gaining accep-

165

tance. Indeed, the whole child concept is not new at all; hence it is not surprising that this same concept is carried over into health.

It should be evident to us all that there will be considerable variation on the degree of well-being from person to person, from time to time in any person, and in the different aspects of health in any person. Since the quality of health, as defined, will be fluctuating, it becomes imperative that individuals be prepared to direct their own behavior in order to maintain the optimum level of health in all its aspects. This gives us the basis for the aim in health education: intelligent self-direction of health behavior, which makes it imperative that we call on every possible resource for health instruction.

Much has been written about the kind of health instruction that is carried on in the health class. There has also been a considerable amount of attention given to teaching for health in and through other classes. However, there is a definite need to give more attention to the kind of health education that accrues from our day-to-day activities, experiences, and situations. What influence does the healthful environment have on health behavior? How can these day to day experiences, often without supervision, be brought to exercise an effective influence on health behavior? How can these influences be incorporated into the regular classroom instruction in health education?

Curriculum planners at all levels should make provision for drawing on the activities and situations related to the healthful school environment in the total educational program of the school. However, it is especially incumbent on the health education curriculum planners to make certain that such activities and situations are a planned part of the school health instruction program. The format suggested for the unit plan may be used in planning for such instruction. The healthful environment is important to the health of the students, but if it is also to provide desirable health education experiences there must be specific plans to make those experiences educational. The following outline is a suggested unit plan for use by the school lunch (cafeteria) manager in conjunction with a selected menu (Figure 12).

If health is fourfold, and if health instruction *is* the providing of learning experiences in or through the classroom or other formalized situations for the express purpose of favorably influencing knowledge, attitudes, and practices that will make possible the intelligent self-direction or health behavior, what are some of the implications for us as teachers?

School Programs Must Be Educational

We must recognize that the fundamental purpose and the primary responsibility of the school is to foster the environment favorable to learning, and *that is teaching.* If education is the function and the goal of the school, then it cannot justifi-

166

Problem Area: *Nutrition*
Title: *SELECTING AND EATING A BALANCED MEAL*
Long Range Goal: *Maintains desirable body weight through balanced eating and exercise.*

Expected Outcome	Content	Methods, Devices, & Techniques	Teaching Aids	Evaluation Procedures
Selects a balanced meal for age, sex, size, and metabolic needs.	Basic metabolism Metabolic needs and activity Food values A balanced diet	Charts showing: Metabolic rates, caloric needs caloric content of foods, and nutrient value of foods. Keep personal records of food intake for 5 days. Evaluate adequacy of 5 day food intake Handouts	Charts Record forms	Self-appraisal Growth records

Figure 12. Guide for Nutrition Instruction Through the School Lunch Program.

ably conduct any program that is not *first and foremost an educational program*. It is generally agreed that classroom instruction should be *primarily* educational, but there is less recognition that the healthful living aspects of the school program should be concerned with education. However, although this is one of the most effective teaching devices, the sad fact is that too often it is teaching the wrong attitudes. How commonly are the custodians included in the planning sessions of the faculty? How often do they attend faculty meetings? Is there any kind of preservice or inservice training program for them, possibly on a county basis and an ongoing basis? How often are environmental problems of the school or community used as a basis for student learning experiences?

Another aspect of the healthful living phase of the school health program that must be primarily educational is the school lunch program. (Note that this is part of the healthful living phase of the school health program and not a health service.) There is no justification for conducting a school lunch program solely as a *feeding service,* especially not as a panacea for poor home diets. If the students must be fed, then arrangements should be made with a good restaurant operator to do it on a mass basis. It will be cheaper, better, and much less irritating to ad-

167

ministrator and teachers alike. Furthermore, if the school cafeteria is eliminated it will free space for about three average size classrooms. *However, if the school is concerned with providing an educational experience,* then the lunch program should be planned and conducted accordingly. *It can be made a real educational experience.* However in this case it may not show a financial profit, which some administrators seem to feel is necessary.

If the school lunch program is conducted as an education program it will entail a number of innovations. Students will be involved in planning, preparing, serving, and cleaning up after lunch. Meals will be served on the basis of their nutritional value, not on the basis of what surplus food may be available from the government. There will be opportunities for students to select from a variety of different foods. There will be coordination of teaching and menu planning. For example, the need for certain foods, such as vitamins or minerals, will be correlated with the availability of the proper foods and alternate ways of meeting the needs will be examined in the classroom. In short, the opportunities for making the school lunch program educational are numerous, but too commonly ignored.

The activities program (clubs, music, athletics, etc.) also provides the opportunities for rich educational experiences in that aspect of the healthful living program. Are there plans to provide health education experiences in the Future Teachers Association, Future Farmers of America, Future Homemakers of America, band, chorus, dramatics, physical education, intramurals, or interscholastic athletics? If not, why not? *What are the educational objectives in these activities?* There may be a direct positive correlation between clarity of education objectives and support of the programs by the administration, the school board, and the taxpayers. There may also be a cause-and-effect relationship. There is really little question but that many of the shortcomings and abuses in the intercollegiate and interscholastic athletic programs, especially football and basketball, are the direct result of having to make the program pay its own way through winning.

The classroom environment provides numerous situations that may be educational, usually incidentally, but if the most effective use is to be made of those situations there must be planned deliberate attempts to educate in connection with and as a result of such situations. Such situations as lighting, heating, proper seating, housekeeping, and the emotional climate of the classroom all provide the teacher, usually the home room teacher, with opportunities to foster an environment that will be conducive to learning about health conservation. (4:267–283)

Students may be given responsibilities for monitoring the temperature control; control of lighting as needed; simple housekeeping chores such as keeping paper off the floor, erasing blackboards, bulletin board neatness, etc.; and for fostering a favorable emotional climate in the classroom through a cooperative relationship.

Effective teaching for health requires that supplementary to the good environmental situation, and coordinated with it, there be conscious teaching regarding that situation. The health class affords an excellent opportunity for using the healthful living situation for and in direct health instruction. Through such activities as planning school lunches in the health class, surveying the school building and grounds for health hazards, a class survey of health practices such as handwashing or brushing (or rinsing) teeth after eating, and planned participation in a sensible activity program for all class members, the health education instructor can use the healthful living situation as an important and integral part of the direct instruction program.

It should be emphasized that any program conducted by the school must be an educational program. Indeed, it is either a good or bad program. The choice is either by action or default. To draw an example from the instruction program in family life education, we either teach for or against desirable attitudes or undesirable attitudes. A jointly planned program, geared to the mores of the community, can be a positive force for good, while a refusal (or neglect) to meet needs in this important problem area results in negative education. The inference in such cases is that these needs are not important and, consequently, they are relegated to the back alley and the dark corner.

If fostering an environment favorable to learning is the first responsibility of the school, then the next responsibility is for the kind of learning that is encouraged. In its report titled, The Central Purpose of American Education the Educational Policies Commission stated that "the development of every student's rational powers must be recognized as centrally important." (1:12) Furthermore, the committee pointed out that rational powers are developed gradually and continuously as they are used in an atmosphere conducive to thinking, [with] rewards for progress toward the goals that it values." (loc cit) Thus it becomes evident that an important task in health education is to foster the development of attitudes that are conducive to healthful living. The importance of teaching students how to think does not negate the importance of giving some direction in the matter of what to think. If this goal of healthful living is to be achieved, students must be given direction in how it can be done, and certain attitudes are known to be basic. In this connection, pupil participation in planning is desirable, but this desirability stems more from the motivation to get the pupil to participate in planning than from the pupil's discovery of unknown or unsuspected needs and interests. If wise teachers of some experience cannot accurately predict the outcome of joint planning, they should reevaluate their thinking. Again, it should be emphasized that pupil participation in planning is important. It is a good educational experience.

The most difficult task in the art of teaching is the management of the learning of attitudes, although cruder methods may succeed in other areas. Since health education attempts to modify undesirable bahavior or to reinforce desirable behavior it must deal directly, but unobtrusively, with attitudes. There is a great deal of truth in the statement that your actions are your attitudes. The impact of the environment on the emotional and/or social health of the students may be overlooked. Teachers who do not get along together, or who use questionable tactics to gain their ends, such as promotion, are setting deleterious examples for the students. According to our definition of teaching, *fostering an environment that is favorable to learning*, such an environment too often promotes similar behavior among students. There is seldom a significant conflict between teachers without a corresponding "taking of sides" by students.

All teachers for health—for example, custodians, nurses, dentists, dental hygienists, physicians—must recognize the importance of attitude development. Neither can they ignore the well-established fact that *what you are speaks so loudly I cannot hear what you say*. In their own attention to health needs, direction of their own health behavior, they have no choice but to expect in their students a very great measure of the kind of behavior they demonstrate. If the mores of the group are as influential as they seem to be, particularly with teenagers, it behooves teachers and administrators to provide the environmental situation that is conducive to good health practices.

Health Education Through Health Services

The potential for providing health instruction in relation to the conduct of the school health service program ranks second to, if not ahead of, the potential of instruction in the various health education courses. The future health welfare of the individuals is closely related to their perception of signs of illness and use of reliable health services, especially their dependency on the medical professions. We often fail to realize the responsibility placed on the individual for recognizing signs of illness, either personal or in members of the family, which should dictate that a reliable medical authority be consulted. With the population explosion and accompanying shortage of medical personnel and services, this is rapidly becoming one of the most important responsibilities of health educators, to teach people to recognize deviations from normal health and to direct their behavior accordingly.

Nature of School Health Services

School health services may be described as those services provided by any members of the school staff that are directed toward *appraising, protecting, and promoting the health of school personnel, and encouraging the correction of remediable defects.* Such services are quasi-medical in nature with the involvement of staff members being directly related to their background of preparation and

170

qualification. All school personnel should be qualified to provide first aid, but medical treatment should only be administered by qualified medical personnel, preferably through the regular channels of the community organizations.

As previously mentioned, Maxwell (2:181-187) has indicated that the basic optimum school health program will provide a happy, healthful friendly atmosphere with a happy and safe environment; a planned and graded program of physical activities; a health teaching program for health knowledge, practices, and attitudes; daily observations by the teacher; an annual screening program with referrals; semi-annual or annual visits to the dentist; and a school health committee (or council) for a school system. With this basic optimum program as a foundation, additional personnel and services are added as the need indicates and as resources permit, as follows:

1. With *minimum health service personnel* available there will be a medical advisor, a nurse (services will depend on her time available to the school), larger health committee, and a medical and dental advisory committee. In line with their established policies, the physicians and dentists will expect the school representatives to take the initiative in organizing these committees.

2. With a *small amount of health service personnel* available there will be added a medical and dental examination on entering school (preferably by the family physician and dentist) and follow up, including home calls from the nurse if necessary.

3. With a *moderate amount of health service personnel* available there will be added a routine periodic examination with referral examination as needed, clinical use of a dental hygienist, and examination of interscholastic athletic squads by school medical personnel, with accompanying interpretation and instruction.

4. With a *liberal amount of health service personnel* available there will be an annual examination of all students and examination on referral, consultants for various health programs, more health counseling by nurses, and screening examinations and supervision of emergency care with adequate involvement of teachers.

The Joint Committee publication, *School Health Services* (3), contains a more detailed discussion of the many aspects of the school health service program. All school health administrators and all school health education personnel should be thoroughly familiar with that publication.

No aspect of the educational program provides more or better opportunities to take advantage of teachable moments than does the health service activities of the school staff: custodians, bus drivers, food service personnel, teachers, super-

171

visors, counselors, administrators, dental hygienists, dentists, nurses, and physicians. In some way, at some time, every member of the school team, including the students and their parents, provides some health services. Such services may range from a simple observation of a sign of illness or simple first aid to health counseling by the nurse or physician. The health educator recognizes the importance of the strictly service nature of the health services, but feels strongly that the value does not stop there.

In view of the nature of the school as an educational institution it is appropriate to question whether the school should provide direct health services beyond provisions for emergencies. Sound administrative policy, as well as good medical practice, strongly suggests that schools should not be in the business of providing health services *except* where the focus of the service is on health education of the individual. If the amelioration of illness or correction of defect is the ultimate end of the service, then there are other agencies better equipped to provide the service. Furthermore, the efforts of the school can be focused more directly on its function in society, that of providing an effective setting for education. This does not negate the school's responsibility for health protection and promotion, it serves to emphasize its responsibility as an institution devoted to education.

The relationship of the student and the person who is providing a health service furnishes the opportunity for teachable moments of the highest order. The old Egyptian proverb, "health is a crown on a well man's head, but no one can see it but a sick man,"* describes our attitude toward health. As long as we feel well, which is true most of the time for most young people, there is no stimulus or no occasion to be concerned about health. But when a person is ill, there is an accompanying state of *readiness for learning* about practices that will conserve health. This is not to imply that such learning is not possible at other times. It is only to emphasize the unusually high vulnerability to health learning of the sick person and to suggest that educational efforts be directed toward capitalizing on such opportunities.

Opportunities For Health Instruction

Health service situations and experiences in the classroom probably afford the most frequent, and potentially most fruitful, opportunities for instruction in health conservation. Daily every teacher carries on activities that provide some degree of health service. The regular observations for signs of illness or deviation from the normal pattern of behavior that are a constant concern for the elementary school teacher provide numerous opportunities for instruction in exercise and rest, prevention of disease, nutrition, emotional health, and/or safety, to men-

* Related to J. Rash by Mohamed A. Allam, a graduate student from Egypt.

tion a few. The regular screening programs for growth, vision, hearing, or general nutritional developmental status provide excellent opportunities for related instruction, whether these activities be carried on by the teacher, a most desirable practice, or whether they are provided by other school personnel such as technicians, nurses, dentists, or physicians. There is urgent need for teachers and other health education personnel, including health service personnel, to coordinate their efforts to the end that more effective education results.

Opportunities for health education are also present in the health service activities of administrators in such areas as planning to provide emergency care in cases of accident or illness, or to provide first aid.

The following suggested unit plan is intended to convey suggestions for developing a unit for use by the school nurse and/or physician in conjunction with the health examination. (Figure 13)

Problem Area: *Health Maintenance*
Title: *SELECTING AND USING MEDICAL SERVICES*
Long Range Goal: *Uses the available medical services effectively.*

Expected Outcome	Content	Methods, Devices, & Techniques	Teaching Aids	Evaluation Procedures
Student seeks medical care when signs and/ or symptoms of illness appear.	Kinds of medical services Importance of early signs/ symptoms Some common signs and what they may mean.	Discussion Encourage and answer questions	Charts	Student expression of interest Student follow up of recommendations

Figure 13. Guide for Health Instruction During Medical Examination

The educational outcomes attained will be directly related to the extent to which pupils, parents, and staff members are involved in planning and carrying out the activities. If the administrator or a delegate draws up the plans, has them printed and distributed, they may provide guides to follow, but little if any education will result unless special efforts are made to study and interpret the printed guides, or policies. When joint planning is practiced much of the education has already taken place before the guides are released. Furthermore, all who were involved in the project are immediately available to interpret and sell the ideas.

173

Unmet Needs in School Health Services

The educational responsibilities associated with the provision of health services suggest two partially unmet needs in this area. (1) All staff, especially the instructional staff, need skills in providing certain health services. For example, all teachers should be qualified to provide first aid, although some will be more highly skilled and will serve as specialists if they are available; and all elementary school teachers should be skilled in carrying out the simple health screening procedures in a manner that will be educational. (2) Special health service personnel, such as physicians, dentists, and nurses, should understand the general problems of school organization, school procedures, and the educational opportunities associated with the service being provided, and they should take advantage of opportunities to provide instruction in health matters at *teachable moments.*

In light of the current trend to use existing community services, such as using the family physician rather than employing a staff of school physicians, this need to take advantage of opportunities to provide health instruction is applicable to all of the practicing physicians in every community, as well as to dentists and other professional health service personnel.

Special emphasis should be placed on the educational aspects of school health services and the desirable outcomes that may result from a school policy of close cooperation with existing community health services. Provision of all needed health services by and in the school may do much to defeat the health education efforts of the school since it does not teach the use of community resources. On the positive side, an effective cooperative program, in which community services are used by the school, can serve to instruct school personnel in the effective use of community resources. In such instances, upon graduation or when leaving school for any reason, the individual is prepared to continue a wise use of such resources. Without a background of such experiences the young adult must go through a period of ignorance, searching, and learning to adapt to a strange new pattern of securing health services.

Three community health goals should be prominent in those set for students. Citizens should (1) *understand,* (2) *use,* and (3) *support* the *community health program. Understanding* and *use* will be closely allied with early school experiences involving these resources, and *support* will come from favorable experiences in their use coupled with the proper interpretation of the role of the resource in the community program.

Summary

Since human beings are prone to accept as desirable the things with which they live, it follows that more actual influence on behavior may result from the environmental situation than from classroom teaching. In a very real sense *every teacher* is a health teacher and *every situation* provides health education opportunities. The teaching may be either in support of or opposition to good health practices. A conscious effort, based on an understanding of what constitutes good health teaching, can produce desirable results. In this, all school personnel (custodians, bus drivers, food service personnel, teachers, administrators, physicians, nurses, dentists, dental hygienists, parents, and students) must share. The prime requisite is that students have the opportunity and encouragement to practice what they are taught.

The effectiveness of the educational efforts are directly related to the extent to which school personnel take advantage of opportunities for instruction in the services being provided, and the extent to which students are using the resources they are being taught to use in their adult life.

References

1. Educational Policies Commission of the National Education Association of the United States and the American Association of School Administrators, *The Central Purpose of American Education,* N.E.A., Washington, D.C., 1961.

2. Maxwell, C.H., "An Optimum School Health Program," *The Journal of School Health,* 20:7 (1950).

3. Wilson, C.C., Editor, *School Health Services,* National Education Association, Washington, D.C., or American Medical Association, Chicago, 1964.

4. Wilson, C.C. and E.A. Wilson, Editors, *Healthful School Environment,* National Education Association, Washington, D.C., or American Medical Association, Chicago, 1969.

Chapter Fifteen
Health Education Through Related Subjects

As has been emphasized earlier, the school health education curriculum has four components: school health services, healthful school living, health education classes, and health instruction in related courses or subjects. While there is considerable merit to the idea that every teacher is a health teacher, there are health-related subjects in which there are distinct and recurring opportunities to provide health instruction.

If we accept the definition that *teaching is fostering an environment that is conducive to learning,* it follows that learning must be the responsibility of the learner. About all the teacher can do is motivate, explain, and present new information or information not otherwise available to the learner. At the same time, teachers should be aware that "rational powers" are central to all of the other qualities of the human spirit. (1:8)

In the attempts to explain the learning process there have been several theories proposed, ranging from the pure stimulus-response idea to the Gestalt theory. Among the theories we find the idea suggested that in some instances there appears to be learning by *insight,* something approaching sudden revelation. However, as Neal (5:375-378) pointed out, such an exhibition of sudden understanding may be the result of previous experiences and, while the step in learning that is displayed by insight is an important one, it is probably just another step, based on previous learnings. As Neal (5:376) pointed out further, learning can be directly influenced by immediate reinforcement of desirable behavior, as proposed by B.F. Skinner, and the element of immediacy is so important that it deserves special emphasis. It is important to realize that we learn in specifics, not in broad generalities. Knowledge is not general; it is an assimilation of specific items of information. This is true even for the so-called whole method. While the approach is with the whole, it still results from a series of coordinated specific knowledges or skills. Therefore, it is important that teaching be done in such a way as to make the specifics involved in the learning clear, whether the method be whole or part. The format suggested for the unit plan provides for a high degree of specificity in expected outcomes and the content to be used in developing them.

Correlation and Integration

While no single theory seems to adequately explain learning, the most feasible explanation is probably found somewhere between the extreme positions. Furthermore, it is very probable that different kinds of learning take place in different ways, for different people, under varying circumstances, and that no single explanation is possible. This is especially true in health education, since the desired learning involves all kinds of outcomes, knowledge, attitudes, and practices. If this be the case, then a variety of approaches should be used in teaching and *correlation* and *integration* are approaches that should be considered.

what is correlation?

It should be first pointed out that correlation *should not be confused with integration*. Correlation *is a method of teaching* that attempts to show the *relationship of another subject,* or problem, *to the subject being taught.* Through correlation, a topic or problem outside the scope of the subject area being taught is brought into relationship to the subject of the course, or class, in such a way as to foster learning in the other area. To illustrate this procedure, in the study of microorganisms the biology class may be instructed in the relationship of health to sanitation, without going into direct instruction concerning health. The showing of a relationship of health to microorganisms, through sanitation, is health instruction through correlation.

The key to understanding the nature of correlation rests in the fact that another, different, problem area or subject is taught through correlation. The biology teacher never teaches biology through correlation. In a biology class, any other subject may be taught through correlation, but never biology. By the same logic, the health education instructor cannot teach health education through correlation, but there are countless opportunities to teach important understandings in biology, mathematics, English, social studies, physical sciences, and other subjects through correlation with the direct health instruction.

The concept of correlation, in which one subject field is related to another subject field, is in direct conflict with the concept of integration, in which subject matter boundaries are ignored. *Correlation relates to method* while *integration relates to plan of organization.*

Two other important procedures for making the school health program educational are sometimes mistaken for correlation. These are coordination and articulation. In reality, coordination refers to bringing into proper relationship. It is customarily used in reference to different aspects of a program at a given time, such as coordinating the school and community health program. In like manner articulation, which comes from articulate, meaning jointed, is used in the health education setting to refer to a desirable relationship of courses or other educational experiences that from year to year produces a course structure that is meaningful to the learner. Coordination and articulation serve complementary roles in promoting an effective school health education program. Correlation is a method used in the instructional program that may be encouraged by efforts to promote coordination and/or articulation.

why use correlation?

If correlation is perceived as just another method of teaching, just as the lecture, group discussion, projects, and problem solving are methods, perhaps it deserves more attention. It is important to give special consideration to correlation for at least two reasons. First, it is a procedure that exists in practice at varying degrees of refinement, and efforts need to be made to recognize it as the method that it is, thus increasing its effectiveness. Second, it provides the opportunity to systematically involve teachers in the health education programs in a manner that gives promise of being unusually effective. A considerable amount of teaching is already being done through correlation, but much of it is superficial and incidental. Conscious planning can make the efforts more fruitful, helping to avoid duplication of effort and possible omission of essential learnings.

Jay B. Nash popularized *teachable moments,* a phrase that has special significance in health education and a special relationship to correlation. The use of teachable moments has been discussed in connection with scheduling and sequence of health instruction, under the caption of the opportunistic plan (Chapter 8). However, the relationship between correlation and taking advantage of teachable moments needs to be emphasized. Opportunities for effective teaching through correlation are at their peak during teachable moments, when interest is high and when readiness is at a peak. This does not preclude planning for teaching by correlation. It suggests that the teacher should be aware of the health instruction potential at teachable moments and be prepared to do appropriate teaching by correlation. For example, the mathematics teacher may use data concerning longevity or frequency of illness as a basis for correlated health teaching. This requires better preparation of teachers than is required for routine teaching that relies on the textbook, or even on the course of study. However, the good course of study will suggest opportunities for teaching through correlation.

179

Consideration should be given to some of the ways in which the involvement of other teachers in the health instruction program may strengthen the program. *Curriculum enrichment* is one of the favorable results of the use of correlation. For example, reference to the impact on history resulting from the disease of syphilis would provide valuable health instruction in the history class and, at the same time, it would enrich the history curriculum. Reinforcement of learning would occur if, in the example cited, the history teacher recognized the health implications of syphilis. Coordination of teaching would result from conscious, systematically planned teaching through correlation, when the teachers involved in a particular phase of the program had the opportunity to help make the plans.

No attempt to improve teaching is without its problems. In attempting to use correlation on a wide scale the problem of individual responsibility looms large. Considerable planning, including the allocation of responsibilities, will be necessary. Care must be exercised that correlation does not become direct instruction, thus infringing on both subject areas, the one being taught directly and the one being correlated. As has been suggested, the use of correlation will require teachers with excellent and wide preparation, since they will need to be familiar with areas to be correlated with their own area. One very serious hazard is that unplanned efforts to teach through correlation may give small immunizing doses of education from time to time, thus reducing the effectiveness of more intensive education when needed.

In addition to calling attention to the need for plans to teach by correlation a word of warning is appropriate concerning attempts to provide all needed health education through correlation. There is serious question whether correlation alone can provide the teaching in depth that is required to accomplish the desired results. Gmur (3:151-157) and Witham (7) both found that direct health instruction in a separate course was the most effective approach. Furthermore, if all health instruction were attempted by correlation, the amount of time needed to do the necessary teaching would infringe on the time needed for the subject matter in the class with which the health teaching was being correlated. This stealing of time from one class might seriously hamper efforts to do a good job in both areas.

The importance of a health coordinator is recognized in all phases of the school health education program. The coordinator's role is doubly important where efforts are made to use correlation as the principal means of providing health instruction, especially where there is any attempt to use correlation in place of the health science classes. The problems of coordination and articulation are so acute and of such magnitude as to require the leadership of someone in the role of coordinator.

opportunities for teaching through correlation

The opportunities for teaching for health conservation through correlation are so numerous as to be almost beyond listing. Sliepcevich and Carroll (6) listed 185 correlation possibilities under 17 different subject headings.

It should also be pointed out that there are many activities and situations in the school program, other than subject areas, which have potential for health instruction. Some of these are athletics, clubs, student council, food service, counseling service, health services, and healthful living situations. Health instruction in relation to these activities is probably more accurately described as incidental instruction than as correlated and, of course, in many instances it is actually direct instruction. In any event, the opportunity to take advantage of the situation should not be overlooked.

In thinking of the opportunities for health instruction through correlation there may be a tendency to confine one's thinking to the secondary school, where subjects are commonly taught in designated classes. However, the elementary schools provide excellent opportunities for correlated health teaching at that level. Because of the nature of the school room situation it may sometimes be difficult to distinguish between direct instruction and indirect instruction through correlation in the elementary school setting. The skillful elementary school teacher may choose to move from a teaching situation through correlation to direct instruction in health science if the circumstances so indicate. Since the same teacher is responsible for the health teaching in that situation, this need not jeopardize the health teaching that was scheduled for the health class. Flexibility afforded by the self-contained classroom of the elementary school coupled with the recognized responsibility of the teacher for providing such instruction provides the situation in which such freedom can operate.

Planned health education experiences must not be slighted. There may be a tendency to become lax in adhering to the content of a planned program when it is felt that the needs are being met through correlated instruction. The important consideration is that attention be given to meeting the health education needs. The somewhat informal setting of correlation may be most effective in some instances, but the informality may result in omitting some important learning experiences if the teacher is not fully aware of what is needed and what is actually being taught through correlation. With an increasingly informal approach in our schools the need for evaluation is accentuated.

what is integration?

In health education the term integration has caused much confusion in thinking. Much of the confusion or misunderstanding stems from its use in other contexts.

181

The term integration has various meanings. Originally, it was used to refer to the condition of the organism in which there is a harmonious relationship of physiological, emotional, and mental processes resulting in a state free from conflict and strain. (4:292) This definition has considerable application in health education. However, the word also refers to the participation of the different races in the same activities. (4:292)

In education the term integration indicates a plan of organizing the school curriculum by combining different school subjects into one unifying project or activity, such as teaching geography, history, art, English, and arithmetic (and health) in a study of the Panama Canal. (4:292) This is commonly called the integrated plan. The term also refers to the integrated course of study [subject] or the integrated curriculum.

As Frazer has pointed out, in the integrated course of study:

pupil activity is centered in themes or areas of living which draw on the content of various school subjects as mutually associated in some genuine life situation. (2:144)

This is sometimes called the fused course of study.

The integrated curriculum is defined by Good as: *a curriculum in which subject matter boundaries are ignored, all offerings of the school being taught in relation to one another as mutually associated in some genuine relation. (4:150)*

The core curriculum is a modified form of the integrated curriculum in which a group of subjects becomes the center of the learning activity. (4:150) It does not eliminate all other subject matter boundaries as does the integrated curriculum. It provides some of the advantages of the completely integrated curriculum for some areas while retaining the regular course organization for others, such as physical education. Needless to say there is ample opportunity for health instruction in the core curriculum approach although a separate health education course may be desirable to promote the integration of health learning into a healthful behavior pattern. This might be particularly applicable in the upper elementary grades and the secondary school.

why use integration?

The opportunities for health instruction are abundant in the integrated plan. Just as with English and arithmetic, health behavior is constantly a part of life, and the wise and alert teacher will use the frequently occurring opportunities for health instruction. This does not mean that planning is not necessary. On the contrary,

182

if the informal setting is being relied upon to provide opportunities for health instruction, there must be well thought out plans for recognizing these opportunities, sometimes called teachable moments, and for providing the instruction suitable for the occasion. Planning is especially important in order that no important health instruction be omitted.

The proponents of the integrated plan reason that we do not live in a compartmentalized world. Instead, at almost any given time in life we are involved in problem solving that calls on many of the skills exemplified by the different courses. When the process of education is approached through the broad areas, the individuals have the opportunity to develop the various skills in meeting the life situations that they face.

Integration of subject fields (language arts, social studies, mathematics, science, and health education) in curriculum planning is one way to provide for the unification of impact teaching (2:11-12), an important concern in health education.

opportunities for teaching through integration

The occasion for using the integrated plan for health education will depend on the organization of the school. In the typical, traditional situation where the different disciplines have their own classes or courses there will be little opportunity for health instruction through the integrated plan. The exception to this is the kindergarten in which the pattern approaches being the integrated plan.

In schools where the integrated plan is in use, including most kindergartens, there is ample opportunity for meaningful health instruction as a part of the activities related to the broad areas of study under consideration. It is vitally important that health be included as one of those broad areas. Under the core plan, health education opportunities will occur both in the core groups and in the traditional courses.

While the integrated plan has considerable merit, it does require teachers with special talents and special preparation and it requires special planning and unique administrative ability so that no important learnings be omitted or neglected. Except in the kindergarten, few schools have attempted it on a large scale. Instead, a considerable number of schools have implemented a modification of the plan under the title of the core curriculum.

Incidental Teaching

In addition to correlation and integration as approaches in health education much learning takes place through what may be termed incidental teaching. Incidental teaching, or incidental learning, takes place when the environmental influences condition the individual in favor of, or against, a particular condition.

183

For example, students who experience the clean, sanitary, attractive environment of the toilet, or the lunch room, become accustomed to that kind of environment and learn to accept it as desirable. Thus, the school becomes a criterion measure that the student applies in other situations. The properly ventilated classroom also provides the opportunity for incidental teaching. If incidental teaching is to be most effective, attention needs to be called to the influential factors and to their health significance.

While incidental teaching is most frequently carried on in relation to the healthful environment, there are numerous opportunities in other courses, and all teachers should be encouraged to take advantage of those opportunities.

Summary

Opportunities for health education in other courses are abundant, whether through incidental teaching, the integrated plan, or correlation. It should be understood, however, that the term integrated program commonly refers to a plan of organization of the school program while the term correlation refers to a method of teaching. Incidental teaching takes place largely automatically, as a result of the environment, but it must have the conscious attention of both teacher and learner if it is to be most effective.

References

1. Educational Policies Commission, *The Central Purpose of American Education,* National Education Association of the United States and the American Association of School Administrators, N.E.A., Washington, D.C., 1961.
2. Frazer, Alexander, "Curriculum Making for Children: Elements and Issues," *A Curriculum for Children,* Association for Supervision and Curriculum Development, Washington, D.C., 1969.
3. Gmur, B.C., "Effectiveness of Patterns of Health Instruction," in Veenker, C.H., *Synthesis of Research in Selected Areas of Health Instruction,* School Health Education Study, Washington, D.C., 1963.
4. Good, C.V., Editor, *Dictionary of Education,* McGraw-Hill, New York, 1959.
5. Neal, D.C., "A Matter of Shaping," *Phi Delta Kappan, 47:* 7 (1966).
6. Sliepcevich, E.A. and C.R. Carroll, "The Correlation of Health with Other Areas of the High School Curriculum," *The Journal of School Health, 28:* 9 (1958).
7. Witham, J.H., *An Appraisal of Health Instruction in Selected Secondary Schools of Minnesota Under Three Plans of Instruction,* unpublished doctoral dissertation, Indiana University, 1960.

Chapter Sixteen
Methodology in Health Education

A number of instructional methods and teaching aids are available for use in planning effective health instruction. As indicated in Chapter 12, methods of instruction must be selected in keeping with previously identified expected outcomes and content. In effect, the expected outcomes identify the *why* of the unit, while the content identifies the *what* of the unit. Likewise, methods indicate *how* the content will be transmitted to insure the achievement of the outcomes.

Methods and Aids for Health Instruction

Generally, instructional methods may be thought of as the delivery system utilized to transmit the content or subject matter of the unit. Assuming that the procedures for unit planning recommended in Chapter 12 are systematically followed, the unit planner first identifies expected outcomes to be achieved as a result of the unit. Next, the unit planner reviews all available factual information on the topic and carefully selects content specifically intended to achieve the expected outcomes. Since the content or subject matter is specifically selected to achieve the expected outcomes of the unit, it is essential that the instructional methods or delivery system logically fit the content to be transmitted. For example, it would be illogical to attempt to teach proper toothbrushing techniques to primary grade children utilizing the buzz session method, since the method would be inappropriate for the content to be transmitted.

Educators readily acknowledge that young people exhibit varied learning styles. Therefore, it is essential that a variety of methods be used to present the content of a unit. Methods should be selected that involve several bodily senses. Utilizing the previous example, a teacher may wish to teach proper toothbrushing techniques to a class of primary children. In such a situation, the teacher may (1) verbally explain the procedure, (2) demonstrate the procedure, (3) show an appropriate film or filmstrip, and (4) have the children actually practice proper toothbrushing techniques. Though each of the four preceding procedures concerned the process of toothbrushing, the variety of approaches involved several of the children's senses and appealed to the varied learning styles of the class.

Regardless of the method utilized, all instructional procedures should focus on the student as opposed to the teacher, since methods are to assist the student in learning. Effectively selected methods should make health instruction a pleasurable learning experience for the student. To accomplish the preceding goal, the teacher should select methods that are at least somewhat entertaining and enjoyable in order to give the student a positive feeling about health. Schneider suggested that:

the true test of effectiveness of any teaching method or combination of methods in health education must always be the extent to which desirable health behavior results or existing patterns of health behavior are changed. (16:146)

Unlike other academic disciplines, health education cannot be effective if health information or facts are merely transmitted with no resulting modification or reinforcement of attitude and practice. Health facts with no corresponding change in attitude or practice are merely interesting at best. According to Ensor and Means:

the meaning and importance of any information supplied to students will affect their behavior only to the degree to which it has personal meaning or relevance to them. (3:41)

In other words, the student must internalize and personally apply health information if it is to be more than merely interesting.

In selecting appropriate teaching methods, attention must be given to factors other than the nature of the content to be transmitted. Read and Greene indicated that:

the maturity level of the student, the time allotment, the materials and equipment available, and the personality and background of the teacher are of equal importance. (14:158)

Though a teacher may know the subject matter thoroughly and may select appropriate teaching methods, other potential problems may detract from the effective-

186

ness of the instruction. Mayshark and Foster (11:255-256) included daydreaming, lack of interest, misinterpretation of information, physical discomfort, reading difficulties, and excessive wordiness by the teacher as potential problems. An awareness of the existence of the preceding problems may help the teacher select instructional methods to compensate for the difficulties.

Effective methods should create a situation in which the teacher provides an environment that enables students to reach their own conclusions. The teacher provides the structure and the raw materials, while the student creates the finished product. Regardless of the method utilized, Cornacchia and Staton suggested that "all activities and methods include or should include some type of discussion." (2:230) In other words, regardless of the method employed, some provision should be made for verbal interaction between the teacher and the students.

categories of method

While it is not the purpose of the book to present an exhaustive discussion of methodology, a description of several methods may prove useful. The methods have been arranged under 10 general categories.

Audiovisual methods appeal uniquely to the senses of hearing and sight and support other instructional methods employed by the teacher. Specific types of audiovisual materials include films, filmstrips, 35 mm slides, transparencies, opaque projection, videotape, and television; tape recordings; bulletin boards; felt or flannel boards; photographs and pictures; charts, posters, and graphs; displays and exhibits; specimens; and models.

Creative projects allow students to engage in constructive and creative learning activities. A variety of the senses are involved, and the student learns through the practical application of knowledge. Creative projects may involve the individual or groups of students. Examples of creative projects include artwork, story writing or telling, construction of models, preparation of audiovisual presentations, and dramatic programs. More advanced projects would include activities such as planning a health fair or establishing a health museum for the classroom or the school.

Demonstrations enable the student to observe in concrete form a concept, principle, or idea presented by the teacher. A demonstration provides tangible support for a concept that might otherwise be abstract. For example, demonstrating the proper technique for riding a bicycle safely would reinforce classroom instruction presented by the teacher.

Discussion involves various forms of verbal interaction occurring between the teacher and students or among the students. Usually, the teacher will give general direction to discussion activities. Discussion may include lecture, question and answer periods, buzz sessions, brainstorming, individual reports, and group presentations.

Dramatics include a large number of activities involving written and verbal communication. The purpose of dramatic activities is to enhance understanding and communication by structuring simulated learning situations. Specific examples include plays, skits, roleplaying, sociodramas, simulations, debates, and puppet shows.

Experimentation provides an opportunity for students to scientifically test the validity of selected health information or hypotheses. Experiments are carefully planned and conducted to ensure the accuracy of the results. While laboratory experiments are often conducted in subjects related to the life sciences, experiments may also be conducted in subjects related to the behavioral sciences. For example, students might plan to be extra courteous and helpful to parents and other members of the family and report the results back to the class.

Field trips allow students to observe actual examples of information presented in the classroom setting. Such activities are often planned by the teacher or the school, but allowing student involvement in the planning process can increase interest in the trip.

Games serve the dual purpose of gaining student interest while transmitting health-related information. To be effective, games should be reasonably simple to play and score. Games may be purchased commercially or constructed by the teacher and the class. Modifications of popular games such as Monopoly, Jeopardy, football, basketball, and baseball are especially useful in creating health-related games.

Independent study assignments are completed by individuals or groups of students based upon guidelines or general directions provided by the teacher. Students are normally encouraged to complete the assignments as they see fit in keeping with the framework suggested by the teacher. Specific independent study assignments include special reading, individual oral and written reports, group oral and written reports, committee work, panel discussion, surveys and interviews, and health practice records.

Resource speakers are usually individuals from the community who possess special knowledge in a health-related area. Use of the right individuals from the community strengthens the relationship between the school and the community while increasing the practicality and relevance of classroom instruction. However, it is important that the teacher be certain that the individual will make an acceptable presentation.

teaching aids

Following the identification of appropriate instructional methods to transmit the content of the unit, the teacher must select the necessary teaching aids. Methods

188

and teaching aids are not the same since methods represent distinct educational approaches while aids are the physical devices utilized to support the method. For example, the use of a filmstrip represents the audiovisual method of instruction while the filmstrip itself is an aid. Likewise, the projector and screen would be aids since they also support the audiovisual method of instruction.

As stated previously, it is essential that unit planning occurs systematically. Therefore, teaching aids should not be selected until expected outcomes, content, and methods have been planned. An aid should not be utilized just because it looks interesting. The aid should be selected to logically support the method being used, and it should have been previewed or tried out.

The number of specific teaching aids available to the teacher is practically limitless. General categories of teaching aids include audiovisual materials such as films, filmstrips, 35 mm slides, transparencies, video tape, television, and tape recordings; pictures and photographs; chart, posters, and graphs; displays and exhibits; specimens and models; felt or flannel boards; bulletin boards; chalk boards; and printed materials such as textbooks, newspaper and magazine articles, reference books, and pamphlets.

Since so many organizations, agencies, business, and industries are interested in health, a large amount of material is available to teachers. Much of the material is provided at a low or no cost. A list representative of the sources available to teachers is given in Appendix B. While no effort has been made to provide an exhaustive collection of sources, the listing should prove useful.

Teaching for Desirable Attitudes: A Philosophical Approach to Methodology

If teaching be defined as fostering an environment favorable to learning, then there may be very little difference between learning as caught or as taught. Truly, the very best teaching is done in such a way that the learning appears to be caught. The important point is that it is deliberately planned and the situation so managed as to tend to produce the desired results. It must also be recognized that, given control over the environment, the development of desirable attitudes is no more difficult than the development of undesirable attitudes. The problem rests with the environment in which the effort takes place and the external influences to which the learner is subjected. The following basic assumptions are suggested because they have direct bearing on thinking regarding the importance of attitudes in health education:

An attitude is what one feels! Such feeling is about or toward something or somebody. It is a subjective point of view, often held without regard to logic.

Attitudes can be developed. We have evidence of the validity of certain principles of attitude development. There is some question in the minds of many people as to whether attitudes can be taught or whether they are caught. It is our contention that whatever can be learned or developed can be taught. According to our definition of teaching it is possible to foster an environment conducive to the development of desirable attitudes. Hence, we have no reservations in speaking of teaching attitude.

Behavior is often the overt expression of attitude. Attitudes and behavior are so closely related as to be almost indistinguishable. As Krathwohl, Bloom, and Masia (10:27-28) indicated, the development of an attitude moves from being *aware* of, or *being able to perceive* a phenomenon, to being *willing to attend* to phenomena, and eventually feeling strongly enough to go out of one's way to respond, organizing these conceptualizations into a structure that *becomes one's life outlook*. This process is termed *internalization*.

Desirable health behavior can only be realized through the development of attitudes that are strong enough to be directive of behavior, almost to the level of the conditioned reflex. When the attitude becomes so internalized that there is little thought or logic involved, the person tends to act in accord with the attitude without having to consciously choose between alternative behavior patterns.

a philosophy of "right mindedness"

It has been pointed out repeatedly throughout the last 2000 years that the real problem in conduct is one of *right mindedness,* of internalizing principles of desirable conduct and relationships. The earlier expression went something to the effect that *as a man thinketh in his heart, so he is.* The relationship of attitude to behavior was well established long before the time of our behavioral psychologists. This interdependence of attitude and behavior is supported by Piaget who said:

> *As we have seen repeatedly, affectivity constitutes the energetics of behavior patterns whose cognitive aspect refers to the structures alone.* There is no behavior pattern, however intellectual, which does not involve affective factors as motives; *but, reciprocally, there can be no affective states without the intervention of perceptions or comprehensions which constitute their cognitive structure. (13:158)*

If, as Whitney (18:52) has said, the solution to our safety (health or survival) problem is right mindedness, how can we bring this about? First, what are some of the traits we want to foster and second, how can we go about getting the job done?

Five traits, traits of right mindedness, which are essential to life as we know it, essential even to survival as a civilization that we hold extremely precious, are being proposed. They are love, integrity, self-respect, emotional stability, and social responsibility. It may be called a list of basic desirable traits.

love

Courtesy and kindness are two of the expressions of love. It involves a genuine liking of or affection for people and has as its basis a love of self (self-respect).

integrity

Being honest with one's self and with others is essential. Shakespeare expressed the basic principle of integrity when he wrote "to thine own self be true and it will follow as the night followeth the day that thou canst not be false to any man."

self-respect

This is closely akin to self-love as proposed by Menninger. One recent investigator concluded that "anyone who has a good opinion of himself probably likes his elderly neighbors." (19)

emotional stability

In his classic book, *The Mature Mind,* Overstreet (12:21-27) related this trait to maturity. The ability to cope with stress and other emotional problems is an expression of emotional maturity.

social responsibility

Empathy is one expression of social responsibility, while a concern for the welfare of others that prompts action is another.

We know pretty well what attitudes we need to develop. Our immediate problem is how to do it; how to get knowledge and attitudes integrated into desired behavior, particularly as it relates to the conservation of health. Whitney believed that:

> the best education is that which, in solving the practical problems of everyday living, also builds up the structure of a right relation to life. (18:57)

While this is true, the converse is also true and the right relation to life leads to the solution of practical problems of everyday living, especially those governed or determined by our attitudes. As will be pointed out later, this belief was supported by President Lowell of Harvard. (1:76) The problem is how to develop this right relation to life. It can be taught and it is the moral and legal responsibility of the teacher to teach it.

To draw an example from safety, if we accept the thesis that desirable driving patterns are the reflections of desirable citizenship, which is normally revealed in everyday activities, then we might ask: Why do otherwise good citizens go to pot behind the steering wheel of an automobile? The answer is ordinarily *they don't!* Occasionally one does, perhaps, under emotional stress or during periods of extreme fatigue or illness, but *not ordinarily.* Poor citizenship behind the wheel is the expression of the real attitude pattern of the individual, and the apparent good citizenship often becomes a front, a cloak of respectability worn to gain favor in situations that do not furnish the insulation from person-to-person that is furnished by the glass, rubber, and metal surrounding the driver. In a similar vein, and related in principle, Walker quoted Dr. Spock as saying:

Teenagers from a truly good home, a home full of warmth and affection, will rarely get into serious trouble. (17:2)

He made a point to identify warmth and affection as two of the characteristics of the truly good home.

The problem of attitude development is one of securing fundamental acceptance, not just intellectual acceptance, of basic attitudes of good citizenship in and for everyday life—right mindedness. How then can we teach for right attitudes? Kirkendall (8:17-23) pointed out that the fundamental problem in family life education, especially in sex education, is that of *interpersonal relationships;* the *basic attitudes,* of *love, respect, generosity,* and *concern for the welfare of others.*

principles of learning apply to attitude development

The commonly accepted principles of learning are applicable to the development of attitudes. Thorndyke's laws, or principles, of *readiness, exercise,* and *effect* are as applicable to attitudes as to knowledge or behavior. Some prefer to use the more modern terms of motivation, participation, repetition, and identification but they are talking about the same things. *Readiness implies motivation, exercise is participation and repetition, and identification is a desired effect.* While these are all important and interrelated, success in any teaching effort consists of getting *identification* (the effect). It is important that the student identify with acceptable behavior, with mature behavior, and with a sense of responsibility for self and others. Responsible behavior is a manifestation of maturity.

What kinds of participation develop right attitudes? The answer is: the same kinds of participation that develop wrong attitudes; it is only the goals and the situations that are different.

Social psychologists such as Kurt Lewin and Gordon Allport (1), studies reviewed by Katz and Lazarsfeld (7) and others, have given us some of the direction needed in our efforts to develop desirable behavior patterns. Studies of the effectiveness of *telling* versus *discussing,* have supported the thesis that decision through *group discussion is an effective procedure in securing change in behavior.* Our belief in the effectiveness of small group discussion in attitude

192

development is supported by Kohlberg (9:129-140) who found that it was an effective procedure in issues involving morality and fairness, both of which have strong attitude connotations.

Studies reported by Katz and Lazarsfeld (7) support the thesis that the old-fashioned method of face to face communication is most effective, and this is a requisite for group discussion. Roper (7:xv-xx) discussed this in the foreword to Katz and Lazarsfeld's *Personal Influence.* We have illustrated his discussion with a series of concentric circles, Figure 14, with influence moving from the few (half dozen) great thinkers such as Einstein in the center to the 12 great disciples and thence out, circle by circle, to the participating adult citizens (10,000,000-23,000,000), then to the politically inert masses (75,000,000), with the few people in each successive stage having personal communication with and influence on a greater number of people in the next lower order; it resembles the pecking order of the chicken yard or the nibble rights of the aquarium. The *personal influence* that the face-to-face setting of the school room or the discussion group provides opens the doors to effective teaching.

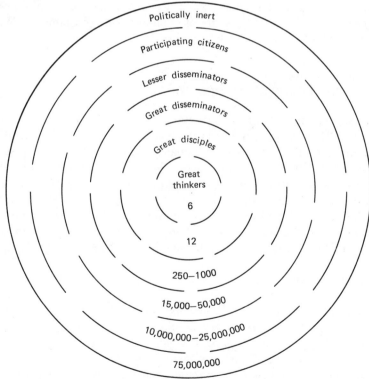

Figure 14. Stratification of Roper's Channels of Communication and Influence in the American Society. [Rash and Pigg, based on Roper (7:xv:xx)].

The evidence supports the contention that efforts to influence behavior through attitudes are most effective through the influence of a disseminator or teacher, on a small group of disciples, and in a person to person situation allowing for free discussion under competent leadership. This principle may be put into effect after the pattern of the concentric circles. Fortunately, the higher in the order we go, the more effective are mass media. The 12 great disciples have a better chance of influencing the 250 to 1000 great disseminators through mass media than they have of influencing the 10,000,000 to 25,000,000 participating citizens.

There is, today, a ray of hope, or note of caution, in that television may open the channel of direct communication between the great disseminators and the participating citizens. If television has given us an effective medium for influencing large numbers of people through mass media, it is the first such effective medium of mass communication.

In our teaching we must remember that attitudes must be built gradually, attitude upon related attitude, and knowledge. We can learn only a little of that which lies next to what we already know. The roof comes after the framework, the superstructure after the foundation. The power of the positive approach must be recognized, and we must be aware of the importance of example. "What you are speaks so loudly I can't hear what you say" is still as true as when it was first suggested.

importance of early childhood impressions

We must be ever mindful of the importance of early childhood experiences and impressions. There is general agreement that early childhood influences have a marked and persisting influence on human beings. In view of this it seems elementary to point out that the *example of right mindedness is the most important single contribution parents can make to the welfare of their children.* Perhaps it is also elementary to suggest that one's family is rarely deceived about the true nature of the individual, and what can be said for the family certainly applies to the schoolroom. *The little day-by-day reactions of parents and teachers do the teaching*—genuine love, integrity, emotional stability, self-respect, social responsibility.

Russell emphasized the importance of example when he said:

both medicine and education have tremendous potential for human good— for improving the function to people of all ages. This potential can be realized as each is practiced by good men and women—conscientious, unselfish, hard-working, sacrificing, intelligent, adaptable people. If practitioners exhibit characteristics other than these, their effectiveness tends to decline and the potential for harm to the culture increases. (15:85)

Allport (1:28-33) reported that in the development of a democratically socialized individual the relationship of a child to its mother in the early years determines to a considerable degree the child's character and mental health. The impact of early experiences was also emphasized by Lawrence K. Frank (4:359), who indicated that experiences associated with breast feeding, the affection and cuddling given the infant, have an important influence on the development of a generous and trusting attitude and are thought by some to be key elements in establishing security in the family group. Frank indicated, furthermore, that when the infant is bottle-fed, the deprivation can be countered by displaying the same affectionate cuddling that the breast-fed infant experiences. This belief was also supported by Galdston (5:11) who cited the World Health Organization pamphlet, *Maternal Care and Mental Health* in emphasizing the importance of the care and affection provided by the mother.

Galdston also stressed the need to relieve conditions of stress that face the individual throughout life. He identified such stress situations as:

—entering school, adolescence, the choice of a vocation, young adulthood, the selection of a mate and marriage, parenthood, the raising of a family, middle years, the "empty nest," retirement, the autumnal years, the senescence. (5:15)

Health educators have the responsibility of helping relieve these stresses through education in each of the problem areas.

In view of the importance attached to the mother and motherhood, it becomes incumbent upon the schools to do more to dignify homemaking as a profession and to prepare parents for the responsibilities of homemaking.

Since the children have established many undesirable health practices before coming to school, it may seem rather hopeless for the school to do much about them. However, since we believe that attitudes and behavior can be changed, teachers must attempt to understand the behavior of the children and then to modify it in harmony with the best information available. In describing the environment that is conducive to learning at the preschool and K-1 levels, we are reminded of the statement that appeared in *The Indiana Bulletin*, Board of State Charities, June 1898, page 19,

It is a significant fact that every vice is a perverted virtue. Cultivate the virtue, and the vice no longer exists. Thus with the child, untruthfulness is usually imagination run riot; stubbornness is strength of will ungoverned by reason. Intense dislike implies intense power of loving. The wise kindergarten will cultivate healthy imagination, intelligent self-control and generous love, and leave the negative qualities to take care of themselves.

As Hochbaum pointed out "if we began to instill in the child proper attitudes and values with respect to these habits [smoking, drinking, and drug abuse] long before adolescence, we could fortify and help them resist such influences later." (6:37)

Allport also emphasized the importance of value orientation and long range goals, their influence on the developing individual and their impact on the decision making process of adults. He quoted President Lowell, of Harvard, to the effect that:

[I]f the administrator is clear in his own mind concerning his value orientations, if he knows his major aims, decisions on specific issues automatically follow. (1:76)

With the importance attached to value orientations and aims, it becomes imperative that schools do all in their power to prepare their students for future responsibilities as parents, and to assist parents in their efforts in rearing their children.

All that has been said relative to home environment and relationships has direct application in schools. Teachers do serve *in loco parentis,* and the responsibilties and opportunities for favorably influencing attitude development should be recognized.

The importance of attitude was indicated in an expression of the cartoon character, The Country Parson, when he said, "Grace at meals is necessary not so much because God needs our thanks as that we need to be thankful."

Earlier in this chapter a number of effective methods of teaching were suggested. It is obvious that not all methods have equal application to the different kinds of expected outcomes and content. Since we are now primarily concerned with developing attitudes that are conducive to the conservation and promotion of health, we will attempt to identify some of the more effective approaches. The use of the taxonomy of educational objectives, as illustrated in Chapter 13, provides one approach. Although that applies more to the organization and formulation of expected outcomes than to method, identification of germane expected outcomes, with appropriate progression, is basic. Methods must be selected that will most effectively translate the knowledge represented by the selected content into behavioral outcomes.

Learning through discovery, as practiced in the HEW (Berkeley) project on smoking (see Chapter 10), has proven to be one effective approach. As students discover new facts and new relationships and, as these are pointed out as significant, the situation is created in which students reach their own conclusion based on sound scientific information.

Decision making through group discussion provides a similar setting where students share opinions, with teachers as well as with fellow students, and are called upon to examine other opinions and to defend their own. When this is done in an atmosphere of searching for the best decision it fosters an environment that promotes the development of desirable attitudes. When a decision is reached by consensus, it is truly *our decision*, with no dissenters. Such an atmosphere might be described as a *meeting for learning*. Brainstorming for new ideas, no matter how "far out," with subsequent examination and evaluation of the ideas can be an effective procedure in group discussion.

In the category of dramatics, *role playing* often provides the opportunity for students to express their feelings without any threat to themselves, and to see and feel how others may react to a given situation. Properly conceived and conducted, it can be an effective method for influencing attitudes.

Resource speakers, if chosen wisely, can be effective in influencing attitudes. Prominent sports figures, community leaders, and health authorities are among the types of speakers who can be effective. They should be carefully selected, and follow-up teaching should be done to ensure accurate interpretations and explanations.

Creative projects may encourage constructive and creative learning experiences in the home, in school, or in the community. These may be individual or group.

In the use of any method, the principle of progression should be followed, moving from the simple to the more complex and from the concrete to the abstract. In order to avoid monotony and to meet the different needs of the children a variety of methods should be employed when possible.

Summary

Methods and aids provide the tools for effective health instruction. The unit planner must ensure that the methods and aids selected for use are suited to the content to be presented. Often, teachers tend to overuse methods with which they are comfortable. Perhaps such a practice is responsible for the saying that *the worst teaching method is the one that is used to excess.* Teachers must continually be receptive to new methods that improve instruction. However, new methods should not be selected merely to provide excitement. A classroom may appear to be humming with meaningful activity when in reality it is merely humming. In other words, *all motion is not necessarily forward progress.* The wise teacher will carefully select methods and aids that support the expected outcomes of the unit.

First experiences; stress, deprivation, unresolved conflict, joy, or satisfaction are so important as to be dominant factors through life. The impact of early stress and deprivation is so traumatic as to be almost inerradicable; *almost*, but *not quite.* Attitudes can be changed, and while attitude education begins at birth

197

it also must continue throughout the whole of life. Modification of attitudes and subsequent behavior, difficult as it may be, can be effected through recognition and application of accepted principles of learning. It would be as difficult to develop systematically wrong attitudes as it is to develop the right.

A positive emphasis on a long range value orientation, concern for the first learning, especially through example, and desirable interpersonal relations provide the basis for right mindedness. This, in turn, will foster the development of the important traits of love, integrity, self-respect, emotional stability, and social responsibility, and factors essential to optimum health.

References

1. Allport, G.W., *Becoming,* Yale University, New Haven, 1955.

2. Cornacchia. H.J., and W.M. Staton, *Health in Elementary Schools,* Fourth Edition, Mosby, St. Louis, 1974.

3. Ensor, P.G. and R.K. Means, *Instructor's Resource and Methods Handbook for Health Education,* Second Edition, Allyn, Boston, 1977.

4. Frank, L.K., "The Fundamental Needs of the Child," reprinted from *Mental Hygiene,* New York Committee on Mental Hygiene of the State Charities Aid Association, 22:3 (1938).

5. Galdston, I., M.D., *Beyond the Germ Theory,* Health Education Council, New York and Minneapolis, 1954.

6. Hochbaum, G.M., "How Can We Teach Adolescents About Smoking, Drinking, and Drug Abuse?" *Journal of Health, Physical Education, and Recreation,* 39:8 (1968).

7. Katz, Alihu and P.F. Lazarsfeld, *Personal Influence,* Free Press, Glenco, Illinois, 1955.

8. Kirkendall, L.A., "Where Should We Go In Sex Education?" *The Coordinator,* 6:2 (1957).

9. Kohlberg, Lawrence, "The Cognitive-Developmental Approach to Moral Education," in Hass, G., *Curriculum Development: A New Approach,* Allyn, Boston, 1977.

10. Krathwohl, D.R., B.S. Bloom, and B.B. Masia, *Taxonomy of Educational Objectives, The Classification of Educational Goals, Handbook II, Affective Domain,* McKay, New York, 1964.

11. Mayshark, C. and R.A. Foster, *Health Education in Secondary Schools,* Third Edition, Mosby, St. Louis, 1972.

12. Overstreet, H.A., *The Mature Mind,* Norton, New York, 1949.

13. Piaget, J. and B. Inhelder, *The Psychology of the Child,* Basic Books, New York, 1969.

14. Read, D.A. and W.H. Greene, *Creative Teaching in Health,* Second Edition, Macmillan, New York, 1975.

15. Russell, R.D., *Health Education,* National Education Association, Washington, D.C., 1975.

16. Schneider, R.E., *Methods and Materials in Health Education,* Second Edition, Saunders, Philadelphia, 1964.

17. Walker, C., "Why Does Youth Go Wrong?" *Guideposts,* Carmel, New York, February, 1958.

18. Whitney, A.W., *Safety for Greater Adventures,* (H.J. Stack, Editor), Center for Safety Education, New York University, New York, 1953.

19. Williams, J.C., "Researcher Says People Who Like Selves Feel Kindly Toward Aged," *The Courier Journal*, January 24, 1958.

PART THREE
HEALTH EDUCATION CURRICULUM IMPLEMENTATION AND EVALUATION

Chapter Seventeen
Planning for Preschool and Elementary School Health Education Experiences

Recognition of the importance of early childhood education and training is not new. Admonitions regarding early training date back to early Biblical times, and there is abundant evidence that all cultures have started early to implant their mores and practices in the minds and behavior of the very young.

It is only relatively recently that these concerns have begun to be recognized as important to the welfare of the child, not just the future of the culture. However, it is important to recognize that these two concerns are so closely related as to be almost inseparable and that the most effective way to influence society is through an effective program of early childhood education based on the needs of the child.

It is also important to recognize that if it were possible to establish the desirable health attitudes and practices from the beginning, the burden of the job of the health educator, as of all educators, would be tremendously relieved. As it is, the educator must devote a great amount of time and energy to correcting efforts. By the time the child gets to school, so much learning has taken place and so many undesirable health practices have become habituated that the task becomes one of helping children unlearn undesirable habits and replacing them with desirable ones as well as helping them learn new habits. To the degree that desirable attitudes and practices are established as the primary or first learnings, the success of the health education experiences will be increasingly assured.

To be most successful, then, health education experiences must be planned and implemented as early as the child can learn. This suggests the need to extend the efforts of health educators into the preschool period in the life of the child.

In planning preschool health education experiences it may be convenient to consider four different stages of development of the young child. These four stages are (1) prenatal, (2) neonatal, (3) infancy/toddler (nursery school), and (4) preschool/kindergarten.

Prenatal Experiences

On first thought it may seem facetious to consider health education during the intrauterine (prenatal or antepartum) period. However, the accumulation of evidence seems to point more and more to the possiblity that the learning process begins before birth. Furthermore, and of supreme importance, such factors as the mother's diet, disease, drugs (including nicotine and alcohol), and stress do have direct and often traumatic effects on the developing embryo and fetus. As Hanlon (5:329) pointed out, to a great extent prenatal educational experiences depend on the health education of parents and prospective parents, since these individuals are responsible for providing the optimal climate for the development and education of the child.

In discussing education of the future Drummond emphasized the importance of protecting and promoting the health of the unborn in order that healthy children enter this world. He stressed the importance of parent education when he said:

much of the educational program of the future will be geared to the solution of human problems. It will start in the prenatal period, with the parents and continue throughout life. (2:35)

Neonatal Experiences

The neonatal (intrapartum) period, that period surrounding the birth, presents many opportunities for the kind of teaching that has been described as *fostering an environment conducive to learning.* Popular acceptance of natural childbirth, the presence of the father in the delivery room, and control of the neonatal environment to protect the newborn from noise, bright lights, and other traumatic experiences indicate the recognition of the importance of the educational experiences surrounding birth. As with the prenatal period, the educational experiences must be directed toward the parents, doctors, and nurses, but the focus is on the learning experiences of the child.

The importance of the environment into which a baby is born was stressed by Frederick Leboyer, M.D. when he said "[to] protect newborn children from fear we must unveil the world to them infinitely slowly, in an endless sequence of severely limited revelations. And not overwhelm them with more new sensations than they can support and integrate." (9:102) He urged that the birth environment be quiet, warm, nearly dark, and *loving,* and that the newborn be handled

204

gently, gradually letting it acclimate to the new environment: new circulatory and respiratory systems, new posture, light, air, the force of gravity, sound, etc. It is this acclimation process that Leboyer believes has such a profound influence on the total personality of the individual.

Infancy/Toddler Experiences

During the period from birth to two or two-and-one-half years of age the child progresses from being completely dependent at birth to achieving a considerable degree of independence. The extent to which the child becomes a happy, friendly, capable, self-reliant individual depends to a great extent on the educational experiences that the parents provided from birth to one year of age. Such experiences include responding to cries; meeting the physical needs to be fed, dry, warm, comfortable, and loved; giving love and assurance in times of emotional stress; and providing an environment that fosters love, cooperation, self-assurance, and self-discipline.

As indicated by Jenkins et al. through such experiences the parents are able to establish a warm and harmonious relationship with the child. Such a relationship is essential to the full development of the truly integrated personality. (6:48)

Since the emotional foundations are well laid during the period of infancy, curriculum planners must reexamine their approach and give due consideration to planning for desirable health education experiences during this period. In the past a few individuals (notably Dr. Spock) have attempted to provide guidelines for parents. Such efforts have generally been commendable, and they will no doubt be supplemented by many others. As this is done, and as better educated parents learn to make discriminatory choices in their reading, we can hope for a more favorable emotional climate for the infants and toddlers.

Needless to say, the kind of teaching that is successful in this period fosters an environment that is conducive to learning. There will be little need or opportunity for direct positive aggressive efforts to instill knowledges and attitudes. Rather, the efforts must be directed at ensuring that the child is exposed to and learns to accept the kind of satisfaction that comes from the care and attention suggested by Jenkins.

Since schools will have little direct contact with the toddler, the only effective approach to toddler health education will still be through the parents. This strongly indicates the need for schools to become involved in parent education programs. Such efforts should take two approaches. First, there must be a major emphasis on education for parenthood while the youth are still in school. Such programs should begin early enough to reach all students before the many complicating and confusing influences of the sex drive take over. Indeed, the most effective approach would be to include planned parent education experiences in all

205

stages of school, beginning with the very simple tasks and responsibilities that may be taught in the lower grades. This could start with care of toys and clothes, helping fellow students when needed; in the upper grades baby-sitting could be discussed. While this may often be thought of as *incidental* teaching, it should be emphasized that *planning* is required to be certain that those desirable experiences will always occur. Likewise, planning is necessary to ensure attention to the needs of the students, those needs basic to being a capable parent.

The second approach of the schools, which is generally neglected, is offering instruction in parenthood to parents and prospective parents. Schools might well be responsible for offering classes for expectant parents, new parents, parents of the preschool child, parents of preadolescents and early adolescents, and parents who have special problems such as drug use, and antisocial behavior. In sponsoring or conducting this kind of education, schools might well serve as the coordinating agency, working with the health department and hospitals while calling on local experts such as pediatricians, obstetricians, nurses, nutritionists, and other health specialists to do the actual teaching.

It is important that these two approaches be coordinated. Either approach operating independently cannot be expected to achieve the optimum degree of success while together they supplement and complement each other. This is particularly true in regard to the kind and amount of support for the childhood health education program that may be expected to result from informed and sympathetic parents of the school children.

There are at least four basic health needs of infants and toddlers, as well as of all children, which must be met if optimum health is to be conserved. These are adequate nutrition, a climate that fosters emotional stability, a balanced schedule of exercise and rest, and protection from trauma such as disease or accidents. Needless to say, each of these needs has widespread implications for the parent and/or the school, but a well-planned and carefully implemented program for meeting each of them is needed for optimum development of the individual.

Nursery School, Preschool, and Kindergarten Experiences

While it is generally accepted that most children will go to school by the time they are six years old, an ever-increasing number are going to school at an earlier age. Kindergarten is fast-becoming almost universal, and with the increase in the number of working mothers the preschool or nursery school is becoming more common. In many instances this takes place in a day-care center; however, a day-care center must be considered as an educational institution, and it must accept the associated responsibilities.

Thus, for the first time in their lives children in preschool or kindergarten come into a rather formally structured situation, a situation that calls for careful planning if the experiences are to be truly educational.

Years ago Lawrence K. Frank indicated the true nature of maturity when he said:

> *Maturity does not mean chronological age or size or weight; it means that the child has had enough of an activity, such as sucking or unrestricted elimination, to be able to go on to something else without a persistent feeling of deprivation or an unsatisfied infantile longing. (3:360)*

In nurturing good habits there may be a serious conflict between establishing good habits and fostering a whole personality. We need to recognize that the development of the desirable personality usually results in subsequently establishing desirable habits. In this regard an old axiom comes to mind. *Every vice is a perverted virtue, cultivate the virtue and the vice no longer prevails.* This is especially applicable in the kindergarten and preschool. Persistent emphasis, recognition, and reinforcement of the desirable behavior patterns (especially the desirable health behavior patterns) will do much to encourage personality development and subsequent behavior patterns that help to conserve health.

The positive approach being recommended does not preclude having essential rules of conduct and behavior. If anything, it supports the need for any rules that may be necessary to insure an environment conducive to learning, which is the prime goal of teaching.

Important as the physical surroundings and overt behavior of teachers and parents may be, they fade in importance in comparison with the emotional status of adults which may be expressed in very subtle ways. Adult expressions may have very traumatic effects on the young child. It is imperative that young children learn to cope with their own emotional reactions such as anger, rage, fear, and grief in such a way as to avoid the physiological disturbance that may often accompany such reactions and that may lead to deleterious overt behavior.

Much remains to be learned about the whole process of attaining emotional maturity, but it is well known that the example of parents, peers, and teachers is a powerful influence in helping children develop a satisfactory behavior pattern, whether it be emotional, social, spiritual, or physical.

As Frank indicated,

> *The nursery school, in close and cooperative relationship with the home and parents, is the primary agency for mental hygiene. The opportunity in preschool education to build wholesome, sane, cooperative, and mature personalities, and to determine the future of our culture, is unlimited. The dis-*

charge of that responsibility lies in helping the young child to meet the persistent life tasks and to fulfill his insistent needs. (3:378)

If schools are to provide the setting that is most conducive to learning several criteria must be met. In addition to a *favorable physical and emotional climate* there must follow the guidance of teachers and parents which will provide *information; inspiration* or motivation; and *interpretation* or explanation. Careful planning must be done to ensure exposure to the kind of educational experiences that will meet the *needs, interests,* and *comprehension abilities* of the students. Furthermore, the *ability of the individual student to act independently*, and the *values of the community* must be considered.

The customary procedures in planning the educational experiences of students will come into operation for these students. Selection of *expected outcomes; content* or *subject matter; methods, devices,* and *techniques; teaching aids; references;* and *evaluation procedures* will need to be carried out with due consideration of the relationship of each of these to the others. (See Chapter 12, "Planning the Health Education Unit.")

As indicated previously, the criterion of need would dictate that students who are on their own for the first time, for example, going to and from school, will have great need to develop safe pedestrian practices. It follows, then, that one of the first formal educational experiences of the students would be some instruction in pedestrian safety. This, of course, should be adjusted to the needs, interests, comprehension ability, and independence level of each student. Community values would not seem to be an important consideration in this area. Some suggestions for implementing such teaching are noted in the sample safety unit for the kindergarten (Appendix C).

Similarly, special instruction will be needed in personal health (hygiene) practices, since this is the first time many of the children will have to be responsible for their own health practices such as going to the toilet, hand washing, teeth rinsing and/or brushing after eating, proper use of tissue paper for sneezing and coughing, hygienic handling of food, selection of food, dressing properly according to the weather, coping with personality conflicts or disappointments, sharing toys and school supplies, etc.

Every teacher will recognize other health practice problems that will need attention. For instruction of optimum effectiveness, the wise teacher will develop a simple unit plan for each area with special attention to the evaluation procedures. The success of any instruction (teaching) can only be measured by the success in attaining the stated expected outcomes.

In order to illustrate the format and some suggested expected outcomes and content of possible units, some sample units for the major grade levels are shown in Appendix C. These provide a model for the development of additional units by interested personnel. They do not take the place of teacher developed units.

Planning for Elementary School Health Education Experiences

Several factors combine to make the elementary school years the crucial years for health education. First, since the attitudes and practices of the children are less well established than they will be later in life, they are more subject to desirable change. Second, desirable health practices that are established in the early years can contribute to the conservation of health throughout the lifetime of the individual. Third, most elementary school children want to learn. This provides a built-in motivation factor that health educators can use to good advantage in efforts to foster health conservation practices. And, fourth, health educators have a captive audience that is amenable to desired results—the intelligent self-direction of health behavior.

With those points in mind it is vitally important that the best possible planning be done to maximize the opportunities for favorable results.

Since, as indicated elsewhere, the needs of students depend, in part, on their characteristics, those characteristics must be understood before the needs can be identified. To illustrate this process, we have gone into some detail regarding the characteristics of the students in the elementary school. Since it is intended here to illustrate the basis for identifying needs, this detail will not be repeated for secondary school and adult students. This does not negate the necessity for curriculum planners to understand the characteristics of the group for which the planning is done.

Planning for the Lower Grades (1 to 4)

Perhaps the most characteristic feature of first grade children is the lack of uniformity in physical, mental, emotional, and social development.*

In general the *physical* development of the six-year-old is characterized by fairly advanced development of the large muscles but a marked slower development of the small muscles, resulting in considerable lack of coordination, especially of eye-hand coordination. Handedness is generally well established by age six and should be recognized and respected. While the brain has probably attained its adult size, this is a period of rapid growth of the heart, which results in considerable variation in the ability to endure sustained vigorous exercise. While it is recognized that exercise will not damage a normal, healthy heart, all hearts are not normal and the diagnosis of defects is not always completely accurate. It is important, therefore, that the lower elementary school teacher be able to recognize signs of possible deviation in heart function and, especially, that these children not be pressured into endurance tests much beyond their natural inclination.

---

* For a more detailed discussion of the characteristics of Elementary School children see Jenkins et al. (6) Lay and Dopyera, (8) Vannier, (10) and Watson and Lowery (11).

209

All "suspect" cases should be referred to the proper school medical (nursing) authorities with proper followup.

Another important characteristic of these children is the lack of maturity of the eyes. There is a tendency toward farsightedness at this age and any marked deviation in this respect should be brought to the attention of the proper school medical (nursing) authorities and subsequently to the parents. While a reasonable amount of close work may be tolerated without damage, provision should be made for frequent change of activity to provide opportunities for resting the eyes.

Children of this age are particularly suspectible to communicable diseases, because this is usually the period of first *exposure* for many of them and little or no resistance or immunity has been developed. A contributing factor, which is an important guide in selecting health education experiences, is the lack of good personal hygiene practices. This deficiency (need) provides the basic criterion for the development of an instructional unit in personal hygiene.

In grades two through four (ages seven through nine), children may be expected to continue a slow steady physical growth. By grade four girls will be ahead of boys in general development. By this time the small muscles are better developed with better muscular coordination, and good eye-hand coordination may be expected. The eyes are almost fully developed and are ready for close work. However, since the heart is still not mature care must be exercised to ensure that the children are not subjected to pressures that might cause them to press for endurance beyond their own capacities.

The lungs, the digestive system, and the circulatory system, except for the heart, are almost mature by grade four. Since permanent teeth are appearing by grade three, special attention should be given to mouth care and especially to the need for teeth to be straightened. A planned program of physical development exercises is essential to optimum development throughout the lower elementary grades.

Intellectually, the normally healthy first grader is born to learn. This is the clear example of the principle that learning is an inborn drive of the human organism. There will be a wide variety in the enthusiasm with which intellectual growth will be encountered. Much of the difference may be attributed to the earlier educational experiences, or lack of them, of children in their homes. Such differences represent one of the most serious handicaps under which the schools must function. If all children could enjoy a *favorable learning* environment from birth, the task of the school would be greatly simplified. Unfortunately this is not possible, so in all aspects of growth and development—physical, intellectual, emotional, and social—one of the school's major problems is to promote the *unlearning* of the undesirable in order to substitute the desirable.

For reasons not always identifiable some children will be endowed with a greater capability for learning than will others. It is the responsibilty of the school to foster the environment that is conducive to learning for all. This leads to the proposal, presented earlier, that there is need to provide the opportunity for *independence in achievement* (see "Ability Achievement" in Chapter 13). Provision must be made for children to function at their own levels and to be able to achieve at the maximum of their abilities. It is in this area (mental) that the criterion of comprehension ability should be used in selecting the health education experiences for the children.

After experiencing the initial mental shock of a formal, structured learning situation upon entering the first grade, the children generally adapt successfully and continue their steady intellectual development. Special interests and abilities soon begin to be revealed. These interests and abilities should be respected and encouraged, but not at the expense of the basic skills. Teachers must be alert for signs of deleterious influences such as illness, family problems, and/or harmful personal practices, such as drug use, that might interfere with normal intellectual development. Learning is still a normal, pleasant experience and any lack of interest should be studied, diagnosed, and remedial measures should be taken.

The *emotional* development of first graders will vary radically. There is very little correlation between physical and emotional development at this age; unfortunately, a child's behavior does not necessarily reveal true emotions. So-called *good behavior* may represent something quite different than what the child is actually feeling and may, in fact, be undesirable. Just as would be done in the case of aberrant behavior, teachers and parents should attempt to see behind the scene and help remove the causes. Children should not be made to feel that their feelings are bad. Rather they should be taught acceptable ways of dealing with their feelings and ways to prevent future reactions that place them in a stressful situation. For example, it is not enough just to teach children how to cope with anger; it is more important to teach them how to react to a perplexing situation (possibly a person) in such a way as to prevent becoming angry. One mark of maturity is the ability to deal with emotions, first by preventing the arousal of undesirable emotions such as anger, fear, and feelings of inferiority and second, by coping successfully with them if and when they are aroused.

The emotional development throughout grades one through four tends to present something of a roller coaster appearance. From the self-assertive, aggressive, competitive, and boastful first grader there may emerge the sensitive, cautious, and self-critical second grader. This same individual may then become a careless, argumentative, accident-prone third grader only to become the responsible perfectionist of grade four, with a strong sense of right and wrong, a strong gang interest, and loyalty to his/her country.

The *social* development of the first grader is closely related to the emotional development, and the child's social behavior will fluctuate in somewhat the same manner. The first grader, however, may be less stable socially *and* emotionally

211

than the five year old. The child is becoming more interested in group activity, increasingly involving children of the same sex. Strong personal friendships tend to appear during this year. The more formal school arrangement increases the stress situations with the resulting problems associated with group interaction.

Throughout grades two through four, the increasingly strong sex identification becomes apparent, culminating in strong gang identification, usually of short duration and changing membership. A sense of right and wrong is evident in grade two. Allegiance to adults begins to disappear in grade two changing to allegiance to other children in grade three, culminating in frequent verbal criticism of adults in grade four. However, this criticism does not remove the need for adult approval.

meeting the health education needs

In light of these and other identifiable characteristics of the lower elementary school children, curriculum planners should next move to identification of the health needs of these children. For example, the susceptibility of these children to communicable disease indicates the health need of protection from trauma (e.g. diseases) and the subsequent related health education need of learning to protect one's self against communicable diseases. One approach to meeting this need is through instruction in personal hygiene; hence a planned instructional unit dealing with personal hygiene would be appropriate.

In planning such a unit, as with all units, the desired expected outcomes should be chosen in light of all five of the recommended criteria. In all probability there will be desired outcomes of practices, attitudes, and knowledge. As discussed elsewhere (Chapter 13), these will be selected so as to best meet the needs of the children. To provide variety and encourage the fullest possible individual development, it will be desirable to attempt to include some of each kind of outcomes. This, of course, will be determined in part by the comprehension abilities of the students. For example, great emphasis would not be placed on knowledge outcomes in the lower grades. Much more emphasis would be placed on attitude and practice development. Provision should be made in the planning for developing many of the desired attitudes and practices to the point where they become habits—habits of thinking and feeling as well as of practices.

The format for developing a unit, Appendix C, is intended to indicate the procedure to be used in developing units along with an illustration of each kind of expected outcome. The progression indicated follows the general pattern suggested by Bloom et al. (7) as explained in Chapter 13.

There will need to be a gradual shift in emphasis on the different kinds of outcomes from grade to grade. The shift will be very slight from one grade to the next, but the difference will be obvious when comparing grades one and four. Again, the emphasis will be based on the use of the criteria in determining what the children need to learn. For example, while the need to be a safe, independent pedestrian was paramount in the kindergarten and/or grade one, by grade four the safety emphasis will shift to meet the safety needs of the older child to include such problem areas as bicycle safety. There will thus need to be more emphasis on knowledge such as traffic rules and bicycle care. (See Chart of Changing Emphasis, Chapter 13.) In a like manner while the concerns regarding personal hygiene during kindergarten and first grade were largely those dealing with cleanliness and communicable disease control, by grade four more attention needs to be given to self-sufficiency in matters of healthful practices, including first aid skills, clothing selection, and diet.

In planning the health education experiences for children in the lower elementary school grades a special effort should be made to suggest a variety of instructional systems (methods, devices, and techniques). It can safely be assumed that no single method will appeal to or reach all students. Furthermore, since establishing desirable practices (habits) is the paramount goal, and since it may be a prolonged task, a single method would certainly become boring to many students. Both a variety of methods and a variety of content are important in attitude and habit development. Thus, it becomes important to approach the achievement of the goal, a desirable health practice, from a variety of directions using a variety of content and of method, devices, and techniques.

Planning for the Intermediate Grades (5 to 8)

It was previously suggested that the most characteristic feature of the first grade children was the lack of uniformity in physical, mental, emotional, and social development. While there may be greater uniformity among fifth graders than among first graders, the fact remains that the development in any grade level, at any age, varies over at least a three year span. In any grade level there are those who are at least a year ahead of the median in some aspects of development and those who are a year behind. This, again, confirms the proposal for *achievement independence* discussed earlier.

This is the period of transescence for a majority of the students, especially the girls. In general, the *physical* characteristics of the middle (average) group in grades five through eight (ages 10–13) include an initial slower period of growth (especially for boys) followed by a preadolescent period of rapid growth in height and a subsequent increase in weight. Girls are generally taller and heavier than boys and are often better coordinated. The secondary sex characteristics, including menstruation, begin to appear in many 11 year old girls. Boys are generally about two years behind girls in this development and, since there is no single manifestation of sex gland development in boys similar to menstruation in girls, it is often difficult to assess the developmental level of boys of this age. The appearance of kinky pigmented pubic hair is probably the best single overt manifestation of sex development in boys. Gallagher has described a method of classifying the sexual maturity of boys and girls based on the development of external sex characteristics of pubic hair and sex organs for boys and on pubic hair and breast development for girls. (4:32-42) Here, again, is a strong case for coordination, possibly through the school health committee, involving such teachers as physical education, science, and health education.

Rapid muscular growth and uneven growth of different parts of the body accentuates the lack of mature muscular coordination, often with embarrassing results. An enormous appetite is often characteristic of students in this age group. A program of supervised, graded, physical developmental activities is of utmost importance at this age. The need to involve school physicians and nurses in program planning is also obvious.

Intellectually, these students are capable of serious critical thinking at their level of experience and maturity. There will continue to be the rather normal curve of intellectual development, ranging over at least a three year span for any single age group. A special effort should be made to encourage the critical reading of good literature and, especially, the practice of written expression. Simple written assignments, completed under the supervision of the teacher, will provide the opportunity for positive reinforcement of the skills of written expression. Small group discussions provide the opportunity to develop oral expression, the ability to think critically and constructively, and provide what is probably the most effective setting for the development of desirable attitudes, especially of attitudes related to health.

Emotionally, this is a period of maturation. There will be a wide variation in the emotional maturity level of these students, both within grade and from grades five to eight, but for the most part they will be anxious to attain an emotional maturity that will enable them to cope with the vicissitudes of life as they experience them. Rapid changes in mood may be expected with accompanying changes in behavior. It is a period of considerable emotional stress, and the greatest contribution that teachers and parents can make to steady maturing is through an understanding attitude coupled with consistent behavior standards and well-defined tolerance limits and limits of deviation. The goal of self-discipline can best be attained through the growing and maturing process, which involves both a decreasing amount of external control coupled with, and dependent on, an increasing amount of self-control and self-discipline.

Socially the students in grades five through eight may become responsible members of their particular groups but there is a tendency to drift away in the early years. Boys tend to be more interested in physically active groups while girls tend to be more interested in so-called social groups. Current emphasis on equal opportunity in sports for girls seems to be producing some changes in this pattern. However, this is not exactly a new phenomenon since in states where girls athletics have been emphasized the pattern has existed for some time. Coeducational sports activities have been accepted in some communities for well over half a century.

As students mature there will be a tendency for the more mature to group together on the basis of interests. Peer group acceptance often akes precedence over adult acceptance, but not without its traumatic conflicting emotions. Adult acceptance and approval remain important at all stages of development. Except for the most mature students there will be little natural interest in dating during these years. It is a mistake to encourage early dating, since it tends to inhibit normal social development by limiting association to a single individual, and often encourages early (almost child) marriages. A varied social program with emphasis on group activities provides the best opportunity for the social development in the preadolescent years.

The warm, affectionate understanding of parents and teachers will do much to ensure a desirable socialization of the upper elementary school students.

meeting the health education needs

In attempting to meet the changing health needs of upper elementary school students through health education the accepted criteria again provide the guidelines. The special needs associated with sexual maturation almost dictate that students be given the opportunity to learn about their own bodies and the changes that take place. This indicates the health education need of understanding one's own body. This need can be met through well-planned instruction that deals with the function and care of the body, including sexual development and its implications as well as emotional development and ways to govern our emotions. While considerable emphasis needs to be placed on anatomy and physiology, this should not be the primary focus. Emphasis should be placed on the health implications and problems of this stage of development, such as acne and the uneven growth of body parts. When knowledge of the structure and function is needed to undergird the desired health behavior, such information may then be added, and it will be more meaningful in light of the problems being considered.

In line with the findings of Byler et al. (1), in grade six it would be appropriate to include a unit such as "Understanding Our Changing Bodies." In such a unit, the desired expected outcomes would appropriately include knowledge of the structure and function of certain body systems, how healthful living practices might influence those systems, desirable attitudes regarding body structure and function, how growth affects emotional and social relationships, coping with peer group pressures, and commitment to desirable health practices. This is one area in which consideration must be given to the criteria of interest, comprehension ability, and community values. Cooperative planning, including students

215

and parents, will be important in launching a new program of instruction in this area.

The importance of including a variety of methods in the plans must again be stressed. Students in the upper elementary grades are capable of doing and reporting on simple research, of participating in decision making through group discussion, and of preparing elementary scientific papers regarding related health problems.

evaluation

It is mandatory that the success of attaining the desired expected outcomes be evaluated if teachers are to proceed intelligently from one level of instruction to a higher level. While this subject is discussed at length elsewhere (Chapter 20), it is important to keep in mind that success in teaching can only be measured according to the extent to which the desired expected outcomes were attained through the planned educational experiences. Other factors must also be taken into consideration in an overall appraisal of the program, but if the expressed desired expected outcomes are not attained, the instruction cannot be claimed to have been successful.

Formats for developing units on environmental health and mental health for grades five and seven respectively are shown in Appendix C.

Summary

It must be recognized that learning takes place throughout life, from the prenatal stage until death. For such learning to enhance the conservation of health there must be planned health education experiences. Such planning must give high priority to the health education needs of the learners as well as giving due consideration to interests, comprehension ability, independence of action, and community values.

Planning for health education in the prenatal, neonatal, and infancy/toddler stages will be primarily concerned with parent education. Schools must accept their responsibility for providing such education. Failure to do so, as in the past, results in seriously increasing the burden through students coming to school with poor or deleterious health habits that must be altered in the process of teaching the desirable practices.

Planning for health education in the preschool/or kindergarten must consider the increasing independence of action of the students and their needs in that regard. For the first time, the school has direct responsibility for health education experiences of the students while they are in school. If the teaching is to be of optimum effectiveness there must be well-developed plans in light of the accepted criteria, and it must involve the cooperative action of both students and parents.

216

Health education experiences that students have in the elementary grades can do much to influence the health conservation behavior in later years. Desirable health attitudes, well established in the early years, can serve to direct health behavior along lines that will result in the conservation of the health with which one has been endowed and which will also promote the recovering of health that may have been lost through accident or disease.

If the school is to meet its responsibility regarding the education of students, then there must be a systematic and continuous study of the curricular offerings coupled with a program of continuous revision of the curriculum in all aspects of education. In view of the rapid changes in the health conservation field it is especially urgent that the health education curriculum be kept current and that teachers keep in touch with new developments regarding health hazards and health conservation.

We now possess enough knowledge to prevent most of the serious threats to health. It remains for teachers, parents, and other community leaders to motivate the kind of behavior that will help realize the goal of intelligent self-direction of health behavior by each citizen.

References

1. Byler, R., G. Lewis, and R. Totman, *Teach Us What We Want to Know,* Connecticut State Board of Education, 1969.
2. Drummond, H.D., "What is Going on in Elementary Curriculum Development," in Frazer, A., Editor, *A Curriculum for Children,* Association for Supervision and Curriculum Development, Washington, D.C., N.E.A., 1969.
3. Frank, L.K., *The Fundamental Needs of the Child,* reprinted from *Mental Hygiene,* New York Committee on Mental Hygiene of the State Charities Aid Association, New York, 22:3 (1938).
4. Gallagher, J.R., *Medical Care of the Adolescent,* Appleton, New York, 1960.
5. Hanlon, J.J., *Public Health: Administration and Practice,* Sixth Edition, Mosby, St. Louis, 1974.
6. Jenkins, G.G., H.S. Schacter, and W.W. Bauer, *These Are Your Children,* Scott Foresman, Chicago, 1966.
7. Krathwohl, D.R., B.S. Bloom, and B.B. Masia, *Taxonomy of Educational Objectives, The Classification of Educational Goals, Handbook II, Affective Domain,* McKay, New York, 1964.
8. Lay, M. and J. Dopyere, *Becoming a Teacher of Young Children,* Heath, Boston, 1977.
9. Leboyer, Frederick, *Birth Without Violence,* Knopf, New York, 1976.

10. Vannier, M., "Children: Their Growth, Development, and Characteristics," in *Teaching Health in Elementary Schools*, Lea & Febiger, Philadelphia, 1974.
11. Watson, E.H., and G.H. Lowery, *Growth and Development of Children*, Year Book Medical Publishers, Chicago, 1962.

Chapter Eighteen

Planning the Secondary School and College Health Education Experiences

One of the most common mistakes made by educators is to refer to students (of all ages) as our future citizens. In fact, the student is just as much a citizen today as is any adult. Obvious differences in responsibilities depending on age and maturity do not detract from the fact that the student is an active, participating citizen of the group and of the community.

Recognition of citizenship responsibilities, especially of secondary school students, can do much to bridge the gap between what the student is capable of doing and what is commonly expected.

Planning for the Secondary School

The *physical* maturity of secondary students ranges from the immature preadolescence transescence of many ninth grade students, especially of boys, to the full adult skeletal structure of almost all girls and most boys in the twelfth grade. In the intervening years there is a wide range of growth rates. During some stage of this period most students experience an improvement in muscular coordination, especially those who experienced an early skeletal maturity. Girls usually mature about two years ahead of boys, especially in sexual development. Gallagher emphasized the importance of growth to most adolescents and that there is a wide variation in the growth patterns of perfectly normal individuals. (5:52-68)

In the early years of secondary school, the heart is still growing rapidly. However, since a sound heart will not be damaged by exercise, and since exercise is essential to normal muscular growth and development, these students should experience a vigorous physical development activity program. A medical examination of the heart should be a routine procedure in the school physical examination and a prerequisite for such a program.

219

Intellectually, the secondary school students have attained a high degree of maturity. They are capable of critical thinking and sound judgment, depending on their experience and the degree of independence that they have been able to exercise. They should be encouraged to think for themselves and to learn from their mistakes. It is the responsibility of parents and teachers to help these students avoid the kind of serious mistakes that would be tragically traumatic. The school should provide an environment in which students can make mistakes and, thus, learn from them, without permanent physical or emotional damage.

Emotionally, the secondary school period is one of extremes and emotional instability. Some adolescents will temporarily regress to childhood practices. The conflict between the need for independence and a simultaneous dependence is confusing and frustrating. Parents and teachers must recognize the strong desire of students to be accepted by their age group, which often results in conflict with parental standards. However, parents and teachers must still be understanding, accepting, kind, and unobtrusive in their guidance. It is important that these students establish long range goals that are value oriented and that schools foster an environment that is conducive to attaining those goals.

Socially, the secondary school student is going through a conflicting and confusing period. Interest in the other sex appears first among girls. Boys are still interested in other boys and boy groups in the early secondary school. First experiences in dating are often very frustrating to boys. Parents can be most helpful by teaching something of the social graces in the home, and schools can use social occasions as learning experiences for the students.

The adolescent is concerned over acceptance by the group, fearful of being ridiculed and unpopular, anxious to establish independence from the family yet obviously dependent in many respects, idealistic, and in need of adult guidance that does not threaten the feeling of freedom and independence.

meeting the health education needs

The characteristics of the secondary school student indicate a number of health needs of that group. Among them are the need for security, socialization, preparation for parenthood, and wholesome developmental activities. The need for group acceptance often leads to deleterious practices among which is the misuse of drugs, including tobacco and alcohol.

The report on the survey of the health interests of students, by Byler et al. (1:105–111, 147–152) strongly supports the belief that students should have a part in selecting what they are to be taught. The suggestions of twelfth graders of ways schools might help them understand themselves and their health were particularly significant.

The health needs can be met, in part, through an imaginative and constructive program of health education. The suggested health education unit on family living and parenthood (appendix C) can serve as a guide for developing other units that may be found desirable in the light of the activities of the local curriculum development group. This is a stage at which both student and parent input can be extremely helpful.

While the emphasis at this level may seem to be on knowledge outcomes, special effort should be made to involve students in learning activities that will help translate desirable health knowledge into desirable health attitudes and practices. Independent study, individual and group projects, and small group discussion are just a few of the effective methods that may be involved in promoting the goal of intelligent self-direction of health behavior.

Cauffman (2:158-174) reported that four approaches were commonly used in the teaching of health education. These were: lecture and group discussion, problem solving, textbook, and audiovisual techniques. The research reported regularly gave commendable ratings to group discussion, either as a single method or in combination with other methods.

As at earlier levels, it is important that a variety of methods be planned so that the varied interests and abilities of the students be met and to avoid boredom with a single approach. A variety of content material should also be planned.

The nature of the desired health education outcomes (attitudes and practices) dictates that few such outcomes can be achieved through a single method used to present one set of content related to the desired outcome. Several different content areas will usually need to be considered, using a variety of methods, to realize the desired results in terms of achieving the expected outcomes.

Go to page 119

evaluation

Since considerable emphasis is placed on knowledge of desirable health practice, there is a serious temptation to rely solely on health knowledge tests as the basis for evaluating the success of the health instruction in the secondary school. Indeed, it is appropriate to use such tests, but they should not be the sole evaluation method used. Considerable attention must be given to attitudes and practices. Attitude scales and practice inventories can be helpful. It should be emphasized that these instruments can rarely, if ever, be used as valid measuring devices to secure data to be used as a basis for academic marks (grades). Their value lies in group diagnosis to determine the success of the instruction as measured by attaining the stated desired outcomes and in their use for self-diagnosis and counseling.

Where academic marks are concerned, observation becomes an important consideration. Observations that are to be used as a basis for marking should be made systematically and objectively recorded. Of course they should be concerned with the attitudes and practices listed in the expected outcomes. Health records may also be used to identify such desirable health practices as immunizations, weight control, dental care, freedom from communicable diseases, treatment of remedial defects, and related practices.

Since intelligent self-direction of health behavior is a worthy goal of health education, the evaluation procedures should focus on the success of attaining that goal in respect to the stated desired outcomes.

Planning for College and University Health Education Experiences

Colleges and universities have a special and unique responsibility in the health education of students. For the first time in their lives most of these students are completely on their own. They are faced with many new situations and many new decisions with new questions that they must answer. As adults they welcome the opportunity to ask questions as individuals or in groups, thus providing one basis for a meaningful health education experience.

As Craig (3:xvii) pointed out, the college or university has the responsibility for providing a healthful environment for the students, for making certain that reasonable medical attention is available to them, and for providing both incidental and direct instruction in healthful living.

The health education responsibilities of colleges and universities are twofold. First, there is the general responsibility of providing meaningful health education experiences for all students. Second, there is the responsibility of providing health education experiences for those students who elect health education as a profession and who want professional preparation in addition to the general education experiences.

While the responsibility for providing the professional preparation commonly rests with the department involved, the ultimate responsibility for general health education experiences rests largely with the administrative officials of the institution. The quality of the health education experiences of student, as well as the health service and the environmental health experiences, depends largely on the vision and leadership of the administration. (6:361–382)

For the most part, students in colleges and universities are *physically mature.* Most of the men and nearly all of the women will have attained physical maturity by the end of the freshman year, if not before. Many of them will not have achieved the coordination and/or strength and endurance of which they are capable. Thus, they can profit from a program of physical development activities, especially one that will have carryover value into later years. This is also a period during which something of a reserve of strength of the vital organs, such as the heart and lungs, can be developed. Properly maintained such a reserve of strength can contribute to the well-being of individuals throughout life.

College-age students have reached their maximum *intellectual development.*

222

They have been aware of native abilities for some time; although many of them have not yet found themselves professionally, that is not a matter of intellectual aptitude but of interest, of likes and dislikes, and the ability to apply oneself.

The tendency on the part of some students to want to substitute artificial stimuli (drugs) for general physical well-being and intellectual effort should be combated with sound education regarding the true nature of the physical organism and its reaction to such stimuli and to sedatives or depressants.

There is a wide range of variability in the *emotional maturity* of college-age students. While it is true that few, if any, human beings ever reach complete emotional maturity, the college years provide a period of stabilization for most students. It is a period of development of long-lasting friendships, including the possible choice of a life partner, which play important roles in the lives of a great many individuals. The health education experiences that are encouraged in colleges and universities can do much to help the individual achieve a high level of emotional maturity, assuming such experiences are planned.

Socially, college-age students are in a critical period of life. For many, this is the first time in their lives they are exposed to a wide variety of socially accepted behaviors, some of which have not been acceptable in their earlier cultures. They are often confused by what seems to them to be conflicting standards and/or ideals.

One of the most important responsibilities of the college and university faculty is to help those students identify and accept the standards by which they want to live, and by which they can live satisfactory, fulfilling lives. They must come to the realization that decision making is a highly personalized achievement and that the ability to arrive at a decision that is not necessarily the most popular one is a mark of maturity.

While social life on the campus often conflicts with the academic program and high standards of achievement, it is nevertheless an important aspect of education. Provision should be made for socializing experiences to supplement the academic program of the institution. This does not imply that the administration should conduct the social activities. Indeed, any attempt to do so would defeat the true educational value of a well-rounded, student-conducted social life. The administration does, however, have the responsibility of supervising such a program to see that it does not conflict with or infringe upon the fundamental educational responsibility of the institution or the mores of the total community.

Meeting the Health Education Needs of College and University Students

The characteristics of college and university students indicate the need for guidance in the areas of emotional health, consumer education, understanding the basis of health and early signs of disease, the use of artificial stimuli and/or

223

depressants (drugs), personal decision making (especially as it concerns health), and personal responsibility in society. Many health education needs can be met through a well-administered, educational, student health service and thorugh environmental health practices and regulations on campus. However, a well-planned health education course can do much to help integrate all of the health education experiences on campus, and elsewhere into a pattern of health practices that can do much to conserve the health of the students throughout their lifetime.

Curriculum planners should take into consideration the possible future health education needs of those in different professions. It might be wise to consider planning health education courses to meet more adequately the health needs of those in such professions and/or occupations as law, medicine, nursing, business, teaching, the ministry, and manual labor. While the needs might not differ radically, the educational experiences might be more meaningful if related to the current professional interests of the students.

The need for professional preparation in various aspects of health and the health sciences can best be met through a professional education program under the direction of the appropriate department of the college or university. Such a program should be planned and administered by an autonomous department, staffed with competent specialists in the field, and planned to meet the professional needs of each field of specialization.

methodology

There is a strong tendency for college and university instructors to rely almost exclusively on the lecture method of teaching. As Dale (4) has clearly indicated, the lecture method is probably one of the least effective methods of teaching while the direct, personal experience is probably the most effective. Needless to say, college students are not going to be led through the simple health practices at the same level and in the same manner that a group of kindergarten children might be led. Nevertheless, there are numerous opportunities for direct health learning experiences at this level.

Among the direct experiences are the experiences of selecting a physician (either a private physician or a member of the college or university health service staff), selecting a dentist, securing immunizations, directing the daily regimen of life (diet, sleep, exercise, etc.), coping with stress, identifying signs of deviation from health, securing the appropriate therapy, and numerous others.

In the classroom the group discussion approach is effective, particularly in influencing attitudes. Individual research and reporting, with discussion, provides an excellent approach. And there is still a place for the occasional lecture by the professor. The lecture is particularly appropriate in areas of health in which there is a paucity of current literature or where research is uncovering new ideas and new facts.

Dr. Marjorie A.C. Young of Harvard (7) identified three of the basic functions of the teacher as inspiring, interpreting, and informing. In addition there is the responsibility of fostering an emotional and physical climate that is conducive to learning.

The small group seminar, of 8 to 12 students, has proven to be an effective approach. Individual reading and research with reports and discussion provide most of the elements that promote the development of favorable knowledge and attitudes that are basic to good health practices. There is abundant evidence that there is considerable value in emphasizing the role of the individual as a parent and the need to serve as an example to one's children and their peers.

evaluation

In view of the widespread use of the lecture method and the inevitable emphasis on knowledge, the health knowledge test has tended to be the instrument or procedure used almost exclusively in the evaluation process. While there is a place in the evaluation process for the testing of knowledge, that should not be the only procedure used.

First, it should be emphasized that the purpose of evaluation is to ascertain whether the expressed desired outcomes were attained, not to just determine an academic mark or grade. To the extent that the acquisition of knowledge is the desired outcome, the knowledge test is an acceptable instrument to use. Since attitudes and practices are probably more important, they should be evaluated. Attitude scales and behavior inventories provide excellent means of group evaluation and of individual use for the purposes of self-diagnosis and counseling. Observation is an acceptable procedure, provided that the observations are made in light of accepted criteria and that the observations are objectively recorded. The Contract for Grade approach has been found useful by many people. As a note of caution, if the contract approach is used it is important that a scale of standards of achievement be set for the acceptability of the work required to fulfill the contract.

Sample unit outlines for grades nine, eleven, and college, are shown in Appendix C.

Summary

In light of the characteristics of secondary school students it is apparent that special emphasis should be placed on helping these students achieve emotional and social maturity. It is especially important that the secondary school health education experiences not be a duplication of the elementary school experiences.

Joint teacher, student, and parent planning can do much to ensure that the needs and interests of these students are being met and, at the same time, to enhance the status of the health instruction in the secondary school.

The effectiveness of the instruction should be evaluated according to the success of attaining the expressed expected outcomes and remedial teaching should be done when needed.

In attempting to help meet the health education needs of young adults, health educators have both a unique opportunity and a unique responsibility. There is the opportunity to work with young adults on an individual and/or group basis to assist them in solving problems they have not faced before. There is also the responsibility of providing meaningful experiences, both for all students and for those who choose health education as a profession.

A special plea is made for variety in methods used in the health instruction, especially that the lecture method not be used exclusively. Similarly, a special plea is made that the knowledge test not be the exclusive procedure used in the evaluation process.

References

1. Byler, R., G. Lewis, and R. Totman, *Teach Us What We Want to Know,* Connecticut State Board of Education, 1969.

2. Cauffman, J.G., "Effectiveness of Selected Approaches for the Teaching of Health Education," in Veenker, C.H., *Synthesis of Research in Selected Areas of Health Instruction,* School Health Education Study, Washington, D.C., 1963.

3. Craig, H.R., "Foreword," in Schifferes, J.J., *Essentials of Healthier Living,* Wiley, New York, 1967.

4. Dale, E., *Audio-Visual Methods in Teaching,* Dryden, New York, 1954.

5. Gallagher, J.R., *Medical Care of the Adolescent,* Appleton, New York, 1960.

6. Moss, B.R., Editor, *Health Education,* National Education Association, Washington, D.C., 1961.

7. Young, M.A.C., "The Learning Process," A presentation delivered to the Kentucky School Health Workshop, Cumberland Falls, Kentucky, June 7, 1960.

Chapter Nineteen
Planning for Adult Health Education Experiences

The responsibility for an organized program in health education does not end when the individual citizen leaves school or college. No other area of knowledge (discipline) is constantly changing as rapidly as that of health science or health education. New discoveries, new developments, and new strains of pathogens are constantly impinging on the current health scene. In addition, the changing nature of the needs of the individuals and the ways of meeting those needs as the aging process takes place dictate that an ongoing process of health education be conducted.

In reference to the needs in health education, Hanlon concluded that:

(1) personal and community health education are fundamental to any public health advancement; (2) significant improvements are necessary in the field of personal and community health education; and (3) the major fault and challenge rests with the schools, health agencies, and the health professions, and far better joint planning and coordination of their efforts are necessary before the current inadequate record is improved. (1:672-674).

Meeting the Health Education Needs of Adults

As suggested by Hanlon, there are three categories of institutions that must share the responsibility for adult health education. First, the schools and colleges have a responsibility for helping to meet this need and their facilities and resources should be used. Adult education programs, ranging from consultant services to institutions and courses, should be available to the tax-paying citizens. Second, the public health agencies (both official and voluntary) should provide services

227

that are intended to be basically educational. These should be in addition to the customary services provided by the agencies. The two classes of public health agencies, the official and the voluntary, have unique functions to perform. Third, the professional associations constitute a vast storehouse of professional knowledge that can be used in community health education. Physicians, nurses, dentists, and other professionals can take the initiative in planning to cope with unmet health education needs of the community. They can also stand ready to assist the other agencies in carrying out community health education projects.

As discussed earlier (Chapter 5) civic and service clubs can be called on for support and leadership in such programs. The vast resources of the consumer services, such as drug stores, which are present in almost every community, should also be enlisted in support of such educational programs. Furthermore, the resources of the sponsored programs, such as insurance company health education programs, should be tapped when appropriate.

It is important to remember that a successful health education program is not confined to the teaching of classes. The radio and TV provide direct access to the majority of citizens of every community. As pointed out by Moss (2:396-406) newspapers, meetings, correspondence, and individual contacts all provide opportunities and means for providing health education. Russell indicated that

three general approaches to education . . . are (1) authoritative, factual telling, (2) charismatic, personal relating, and (3) active involvement of people in the learning process. (3:236)

These approaches are not limited to use in the classroom. In fact, they are probably more applicable in the voluntary program in the community than they are in the classroom. There are numerous opportunities for adult health education through organized groups that may already be functioning in the community, through school and community health councils, and through the encouragement of people not reached in this manner to come together around common interests. Only through a cooperative program involving all of the potential health and education agencies of the community can the changing needs of health education be met.

Hanlon (1:672-674) suggested that there are five phases of activities in public health education: *analysis, sensitization, publicity, education*, and *motivation*.

Analysis includes a study of the problems of the community (or individual), the factors that generated the problems, and the characteristics of individuals or groups involved. *Sensitization* involves all the measures that will alert the citizens to the problems and measures that are being taken to solve them. *Publicity* is closely related to sensitizing, but it provides more details on the sensitizing procedures, including related information. *Education* consists of the procedures to provide the basis for learning, such as providing information. It takes place in a rather intimate manner involving personal contact between the learner and the educator. *Motivation* is the force that translates knowledge into action. In this respect the health educator serves as a catalyst. In planning the health education curriculum for adults, these phases must be given appropriate consideration.

Perhaps the most significant characteristic of the adult population is that it comprises a diverse and changing group. There could be many approaches to classifying the adult population, but for our purpose, that of providing a basis for planning a health education curriculum, three broad classifications will be considered. These are young adults, the middle years, and retirement.

young adults

For purposes of curriculum planning the classification of young adults includes all people who are out of school, on their own, who are generally involved in establishing themselves in their chosen profession, and who are involved in establishing a home and probably rearing a family. The age range may be from 16 to 35 or 40.

This category includes the period during which the violent death rate is highest, maternal deaths are most common, the incidence of mental illness (including alcoholism) is high, and parents are concerned with the many problems of child rearing. These health problems indicate the need for certain specific kinds of health education.

Schools and colleges can assist the young adult population in meeting and solving many of these health problems by furnishing opportunities for health education through adult education programs. To counter the high mental illness and violent death rates, various educational programs may be offered that deal with safety, emotional problems, family stability, and emergency medical care. Parents and prospective parents can be offered educational opportunities concerning the need for prenatal medical care, the influence of the health of the mother on her unborn child, the rearing of children, and meeting health emergencies in the home.

middle years

In the years between about age 40 and retirement at about 65, one of the most serious problems, especially in men around age 40, is the sudden and often fatal heart attack. In addition, those in the middle years are beginning to experience a marked increase in the appearance of the symptoms of arthritis and other chronic and debilitating deseases. The late middle years, age 50 to 65, are often dubbed the proverbial age of the 4 Bs (bald, bifocals, bulging, and bilious).

In the area of mental health, the late middle years carry with them the prob-

229

lems of the empty nest, when the children are out on their own and away from home. This experience is often most traumatic for the wife and mother. It is also the period when the wage earner becomes overly concerned with his or her success in work, with the accompanying stresses.

Since the chronic diseases, especially those that develop slowly, will be showing their first signs and symptoms it is very important that persons of this age be able to recognize the first signs of deviation from health. Early detection and diagnosis are most important for such diseases as cancer, high blood pressure (hypertension), arteriosclerosis (hardening of the arteries), atheroselerosis (deposit of cholesterol on the artery walls), and arthritis. In many cases, early medical attention can result in a complete cure and a normal maximum life expectancy. In any case, the possibility of controlling the condition is enhanced through early medical care.

Since many of the conditions are related to obesity, special attention should be given to nutrition in the aging population and to the relationship of overweight to those diseases. Also, since the first signs of disease are often insidious and not readily recognized, individuals must be instructed in recognizing those signs. This indicates the need for special instruction in recognizing the early signs of disease.

While the primary responsibility for health education for adults may seem to rest with the public health agencies, the school is still the recognized educational agency in the community, and school participation in such a program may reap dividends in community good will and support that can have far reaching results. Working cooperatively with the community health educator and representatives of business and industry, a plan can be developed in which the school provides the facilities while various official and voluntary health agencies supply the personnel leadership. This is the period in life in which emphasis should be placed on preparation for retirement.

retirement

Two factors work together to compound the health problems during retirement. First is the natural aging process and the various health problems that tend to accompany it. Second is the drastic change in the life style that results from giving up the job. This change is often the most traumatic experience and, as a result, it tends to complicate other health problems.

The problems associated with retirement will be avoided, or at least minimized, if the health education agencies have met their responsibilities during the earlier years. This should by all means have included extensive preparation for retirement. However, in spite of a good background for retirement, health problems will arise.

The first health problem of the retiree and spouse is to face a changed lifestyle. The presence of the retiree in the home all day may be a problem to many,

230

both the former worker and the homemaker. A well-planned educational program that focuses on the problems of retirement can serve two purposes. First, it can provide the retired couple with activities that help prevent the monotony of just being at home. In addition, it can assist the retiree in meeting the prevailing health needs through education on the problems of what to look for and how to satisfy them.

Prominent among the health problems of the retiree is nutrition. It is important that the elderly maintain good nutrition. This includes a concern for weight control. A nutrition class that may meet in the school building can focus on the problems of the retiree, for example, how to shop economically. Needless to say, it is important that both members of the family be involved, with due consideration for the responsibilities of each. This is an area in which the resources of consumer services (such as drug and grocery stores) can be involved. For example, the nutrition consultant employed by the food store may serve as the instructor or resource person for the class.

The area of mental health provides numerous opportunities for health education. In addition to adjusting to retirement, there are problems such as adjusting to the limitations of aging, coping with the death of family and friends, adjusting to being single, and worry over finances, especially health care.

Other health problems that merit special consideration include the need for meeting medical emergencies (first aid or emergency medical care); early recognition of the need for medical care, including dental care; problems associated with financing medical care, including the role of medicare, medicaid, and health insurance plans; types of health care including home care by visiting nurses, hospitalization, nursing homes, and retirement communities; and, especially important, a hygienic regimen of exercise and rest.

In planning the health education curriculum for any group it is important to include members of that group in the planning body. It is especially important that representatives of these adult groups be involved in the planning. Thus, the curriculum development committee for these groups should include wide representation from the group for which the planning is being done. Such representation serves the dual role of providing input from those concerned and of serving as a line of communication between the planners and the consumers. Thus, it provides the opportunity to recruit the participation of those most in need of the education.

Evaluation

As with any evaluation, the true measure of the success of the program will be the extent to which the health practices of the individuals are improved. This can best be determined by the group itself. Since no marks or grades will be involved, the evaluation can really be focused on the results as observed or reported, or as re-

231

flected in improved health practices and the effect on the health of the individuals. Reports of how emergencies have been met, of weight control, and of experiences with home health care, for example, can provide objective evidence of the degree of success of the program.

One approach to evaluation would be to have a short feedback and evaluation period during each class session, either at the beginning or end of the class. Another approach would be to devote one session to an evaluation of the classes. A combination of these two approaches might be even more effective.

It is important that an effort be made to appraise the effectiveness of the health education efforts and that the participants, the consumers, be included in the process.

The sample units that we have prepared for adults, Appendix C, are intended to suggest the kinds of units that may be used with this population group. Health educators are urged to enlist the cooperation of adults in developing additional units.

Summary

Secondary schools and institutions of higher learning share with public health agencies the responsibility for the continuing health education of the public.

The adult population falls rather logically into three age groups: the young adults, the middle years, and retirement. Each of these groups has special health education needs that can be met through an ongoing program of health education.

Evaluation of the success of such a program is an essential part of the program, and participation in such an evaluation might well be the most important aspect of the total experience.

References

1. Hanlon, J.J., *Public Health Administration and Practice*, Mosby, St. Louis, 1974.
2. Moss, B.R., Editor, *Health Education*, National Education Association, Washington, D.C., 1961.
3. Russell, R.D., *Health Education*, A project of the Joint Committee on Health Problems in Education of the National Education Association and the American Medical Association, National Education Association, Washington, D.C., 1975.

Chapter Twenty
Appraising Health Education*

Numerous approaches have been proposed for evaluating the school health education program. Beauchamp (4) proposed evaluating the curriculum on the basis of the use of the curriculum guide, Goodlad (5) recommended that new programs be evaluated on the basis of student performance and opinion, while Rash and others (11) proposed evaluating the total school health program on the basis of the availability and apparent quality of facilities and programs.

Beauchamp indicated that there are three concerns in curriculum evaluation:

(1) Do teachers actually use the curriculum guide for instructional planning? (2) Is the curriculum effective in predicting the achievement of the students in accordance with the stated aims or purposes? and (3) Does the evaluation influence subsequent planning? (4:177)

Goodlad suggested four different means of evaluating new programs: (1) Observation of whether or not the students for whom the material is intended appear to be progressing successfully; (2) both casual and systematic questioning of students involved in the programs; (3) periodic examination of students by tests designed to cover the new material; and (4) comparative testing of students in the new and the old programs with traditional and specially designed tests. (5:98–99).

Means reported that one of the earliest studies to evaluate the effects of health instruction was begun in 1921, in Malden, Massachusetts. It encompassed grades four through six and carried these children through three succeeding

---

* This chapter is based on an article by Rash that was published in *The Journal of School Health*, 23, 1 and 23, 2 (1953). Used with the permission of The American School Health Association.

grades. The director of the study, C.E. Turner, reported that "definite improvements in health habits were shown." (7:89) The study culminated in the publication of the *Malden Health Series*, the first health education series with a specific book for each grade.

Pigg (9) identified over 60 instruments for use in evaluating the school health program. He found that recent activities to evaluate health instruction programs "have been concerned with either (1) evaluating the effectiveness of health instruction by assessing the level of health education of public school students, or (2) developing instruments or criteria by which the health instruction program may be evaluated as one area of the total school health program." (10:585–586) One of the instruments he identified was a Score Card, which was developed by Patty and refined by Rash (11). It was designed for use in appraising the total school health program, through an evaluation of the number and apparent quality of the facilities and services present in the school. These were considered under the four main headings of administration and coordination, health services, healthful environment, and health instruction. Each individual item was assigned a maximum possible score against which the individual members of a skilled evaluation team of three or five members judged the item. The median score of the team was used as the best representation of the quality of the item. Subsequent recommendations regarding program improvement were based on the scores of the individual items. In spite of the obvious weakness of subjective judgments by the evaluators, in practice this score card has been found to be a useful instrument in securing data to be used as a basis for recommending improvements in the school health program.

Anderson (2) developed an evaluation scale along the same lines as the scale developed by Patty. He also reported success in using the scale. Wilson (15) developed a scale for evaluating the health instruction in secondary schools. It was modeled after the Patty-Rash scale. One of the most significant aspects of the scale was a procedure for use in evaluating teacher effectiveness as judged by the teacher and the evaluators.

The health education curriculum committee should exercise the responsibility of making the appropriate evaluations. It may be desirable to delegate this responsibility to appropriate subcommittees, which are more directly concerned with the aspects being evaluated, such as the health services department, the environmental health division, and the health education department. In any event, the report of the evaluation committee should be made to the curriculum committee, and appropriate steps should be taken to followup the recommendations of the evaluative body. While the concerns expressed by Beauchamp and Goodlad may appear to apply only to the instructional program, if all aspects of the school health program are to contribute to the optimal health educational development of the students the other aspects must also be evaluated. Such evaluations will be in terms of the goals set for each division. For example, are the students attaining the optimal educational benefits from their experiences in the school health services, or from their environmental health experiences?

Since the health education course of study, the health class(es), constitute(s) the heart of the school health education program, major consideration is being given to the evaluation of the results of the instructional program.

In addition to the concerns expressed by Beauchamp (4:177) and Goodlad (5:98–99), another vital concern is, are the students achieving the expected outcomes stated in the unit plans of the course of study? The answer to this question provides some of the data that can be used to evaluate the instructional program.

In the development of instructional units in health education the focus of attention is on expected outcomes. In the light of the pupil's needs, interests, comprehension ability, and dependency (ability to act independently) the desired outcomes are selected, with due consideration for community values. The further development of the unit relates directly to these expected outcomes. Content, methods and devices, teaching aids, references, and evaluation procedures are all geared to the expected outcomes.

Success in teaching is measured according to the attainment of the expected outcomes. The purpose of evaluation is to be able to appraise the success of teaching in terms of achieving the expressed expected outcomes. It is not sufficient to be able to point to some outcomes that resulted from the experience. Unless a fair proportion of the *expected outcomes* are realized there is reason to feel that the teaching has not been effective. It is inevitable that there be some outcomes from any experience. However, the *purpose of instruction is to facilitate the attainment of desired outcomes.* Hence, it is imperative that we be able to appraise the extent to which teaching is effective. To this end effective evaluation procedures must be suggested in relation to the outcomes desired.

Tests, Measurements, and Evaluation

It is important to distinguish between testing, measuring, and evaluating. *Test* as used in psychology is defined as "a standardized procedure for eliciting responses upon which appraisal of the individual can be based." (3:1251) *Measure* is defined as the "act or process of ascertaining the extent, dimensions, quantity, etc., of something by comparison with a standard." (3:755) *Evaluate* is defined as "to ascertain the value or amount of; appraise carefully." (3:415)

According to these definitions, testing elicits a response that may be compared to a standard to determine the value. This is the concept of the relationship of testing, measuring, and evaluating that will be used in this discussion. Appraisal is the use of the procedures of *testing, measuring*, and *evaluating* to determine the success of attaining the desired outcomes. Appraisal is a procedure in-

235

volving collection of data, critical analysis, comparisons, and judgmental decisions based on the available data. The final stages of the procedure became largely a process of logic, which cannot be reduced to a set formula, or a set of formulas, that will be applicable to all situations. Since it invoves qualitative data, it becomes a process of critical analysis that must depend on or be related to the purposes of health education as set forth in the statements of expected outcomes.

Testing is not limited to collecting data by means of the paper and pencil test. In a very real sense observation of behavior may be thought of as a test. So, also, may a study of the health records of a student to determine whether immunizations are being kept up to date or whether the recommended health or medical measures have been carried out. In short, any procedure that is carried out to gather information upon which an appraisal of an individual can be made is considered to be a test.

The process of evaluation in health education is complicated by the diversity of kinds of outcomes and the problems associated with testing and measuring knowledges, attitudes, and practices. It is further complicated by the need for expressing the results of the evaluation in terms of an academic mark or grade. Procedures applicable in one area of outcomes, such as knowledges, are not applicable in another area, such as attitudes, especially when an academic mark must be determined through the process.

It is readily apparent that a variety of procedures must be called into use if the diverse outcomes of health education are to be appraised in a valid, reliable, and objective manner. Procedures that may be valid and reliable for use in evaluating for counseling purposes or for self-evaluation may become invalid when used as a basis for determining academic marks. The attitude scale is a good example. A student may willingly and honestly reveal his attitude when an academic mark is not at stake, but he may immediately, and to a degree unconsciously, withhold his true attitude if a mark is involved and instead of revealing his attitude he may give the response he believes to be the one desired. He may even be very reliable in such responses, but they are not valid responses. It behooves the instructor to understand the appropriate uses of the various tests, scales, inventories, etc., and to use them accordingly.

Kinds of Tests

Some of the common procedures used as a basis of securing data to be used in the evaluation include tests, scales, inventories, health records, and observations. *Tests* will ordinarily be health knowledge tests, either short answer or essay. *Scales* will ordinarily be attitude scales. *Inventories* will ordinarily be practice or behavior inventories. *Health records* may reveal practices regarding medical and dental examinations, immunizations, dental care, growth, nutritional status, corrections of defects or handicaps, and preventable illnesses. *Observation* may be valuable in evaluating attitudes and practices in the area of mental health or human relations as well as in common hygienic practices such as covering coughs and sneezes, cleanliness, posture, etc.

The traditional paper and pencil tests have furnished the basis for much of the evaluation that has been attempted in the past. Other methods include recorded observation by teacher and parent; personal inventory, such as practice or habit inventories; pupil and parent questionnaires; self-evaluation scales; and the like. However, in the area of health and health education the paper and pencil tests continue to occupy a position of considerable importance in the evaluation program. This is particularly true in the higher grades, junior and senior high school, and college, where health knowledge justifiably receives major attention. These paper and pencil tests have taken various forms, ranging from the traditional discussion question to the highly refined short answer, or objective test, and covering at least two types of learning—knowledges, and attitudes.

Various attempts to arrive at valid, reliable, and objective data have resulted in tests ranging from those consisting of elements of a single type to those made up of a battery of tests. There have been few attempts to measure health practices by means of the paper and pencil tests. Perhaps it is also worthy of note that authors of the health attitude tests, or scales, warn specifically against using the results of these tests as a basis for marking. However, it is important that school people in particular not limit their conception of the term evaluation to marking purposes. One of the principal functions of tests, as pointed out by Patty (8:68–63) is to improve learning for health. Efforts to improve learning for health will involve at once the evaluation of teaching as well as the evaluation of learning. The extent to which the expected outcomes do appear as outcomes will bear a very close relationship to the effectiveness of the teaching. To this extent, then, an evaluation of outcomes becomes, in reality, an appraisal of teaching.

If it is intended that paper and pencil tests (particularly short answer tests) may serve as an important tool in the whole appraisal process, it becomes important that these tests be as valid, reliable, and objective as it is possible to make them. A number of selected health knowledge tests are included in Appendix B. Individuals interested in a detailed listing of evaluation instruments may wish to consult *Evaluation Instruments in Health Education* compiled by Marion K. Solleder and available from the American Alliance for Health, Physical Education and Recreation in Washington, D.C.

There seems to be a widespread failure to recognize the importance of objectivity, validity, and reliability in using observations as a method of securing data. It is important that the observations be made systematically, specific for desired outcomes, according to established and uniform standards, and that they be objectively recorded. It would seem to be desirable for an elementary teacher, for example, to observe a few pupils for a well-defined expected outcome for an extended period of time and that the results be recorded for future reference. By observing small sections of a class in this manner for a specified period of time, the teacher could observe the entire class in a few days. Failure to keep accurate records of observations tends to invalidate observations as a desirable procedure for securing the data to be used in the evaluation process.

Constructing Health Education Tests

As we have emphasized, evaluation in health education involves considerably more than testing. However, since testing is one of the important procedures for use in such evaluation, we have included some suggestions regarding the construction and use of tests. For a more detailed treatment of test construction the reader is referred to Thorndike and Hagen. (13) The chapter on locally constructed tests (13:198–272) will be particularly helpful to the teacher who is concerned with constructing health education tests. We will discuss the main steps in constructing a test. It is generally agreed that the seven distinct steps in developing a refined test are: (1) Determine instructional objectives, or outcomes to be tested. (2) Prepare a table of specifications, or test outline, in harmony with the instructional objectives and emphasis (balance). (3) Prepare test items in harmony with the table of specifications. (4) Prepare directions, key, and arrange the mechanical features of the test. (5) Administer the trial application. (6) Refine the test in light of the results of the trial application. (7) Administer the refined test.

The commonly recognized criteria for test construction are validity, reliability, and obectivity. Stated simply, *validity* means that the test measures what it purports to measure; *reliability* means it measures consistently what it does measure; and *objectivity* means there is reliability (consistency) of scoring. It is also claimed that administrability, economy, and interpretability are criteria worthy of consideration. *Administrability* means it can be administered readily; *economy* means it is not expensive of time or money; and *interpretability* means the test results have, or can be made to have, meaning in the situation.

instructional objectives

As already emphasized, evaluation in health education must be in relation to instructional objectives. These will be in the areas of knowledges, attitudes, and practices and the test, scale, or inventory must of necessity be in harmony with the kinds of outcomes to be evaluated. Furthermore, there must be specificity of test items in relation to expected outcomes.

balance

A table of specifications should be drawn up that will be in harmony with the emphasis of the expected outcomes. This should indicate the number of each kind of test items to be developed and the proportion of the total test items to be devoted to each instruction area. The more important expected outcomes, both in terms of time devoted and cruciality of the outcome, will be allocated an appropriate proportion of the test items. A table of specifications furnishes a guide to the test constructor in developing test items. One should not be expected to follow it to the exact figure, since some outcomes lend themselves more readily to being evaluated. Some of the most important outcomes are difficult to test and, hence, the balance may not be in exact proportion to the objectives. However, the table of specifications is a valuable guide, particularly for developing a standardized test over a large subject matter area.

test items

The ultimate key to the quality of the test is the test item. Some of the more common kinds of objective test items are the true-false, multiple choice, best answer, matching, corrected true-false, and completion.

Health educators should not overlook the values of the essay or discussion test. A well-formulated essay question can elicit an in-depth response that can reveal the knowledge and attitudes of the respondent and at the same time provide an exercise in logical thinking and expression that are essential elements in anyone's education.

In practical application the valid health knowledge test elicits a response, which may be compared to a standard to determine the value in terms of health knowledge. In similar manner the valid attitude scale and the valid practice inventory make it possible to determine a value for attitudes and practices, respectively. If the tests are consistent in this regard they may be said to be reliable.

The significance of these facts, in relation to unit planning, lies in the need to select and use tests that do actually make it possible to evaluate the effectiveness of instruction intended to secure an expected outcome.

Since the details of test construction are beyond the scope of this book, suffice it to say the multiple choice item is generally thought to be the best single kind of item for testing knowledge, attitudes, and practices where the material lends itself to that kind of item. However, for certain kinds of materials it is not possible to provide four or five plausible options; therefore the alternative is often to use another kind of item, probably the true-false. Whereas the single true-false test item is usually thought to be relatively low in reliability, this is compensated for in part by the ability to test a broad area of knowledge in a short time. The matching items are very satisfactory for certain kinds of health information. While the steps indicated above have a more direct application in constructing the short answer tests, they also have application to the essay test. For example, the essay test should be directed toward the instructional objectives, and the table of specifications should indicate the emphasis to be given to different aspects of the material to be tested. Also, the directions should be specific regarding the emphasis considered to be important. A scoring key should reflect the emphasis desired, while trial application, refinement, and use of the test will correspond to the same steps as for a short answer test.

Since the scoring of an essay test is generally thought to be less reliable than for short answer tests, it is important that the procedure be as objective as possible. The objectivity can be increased by using a key that indicates subjects to be discussed and the relative point value of those subjects. The authors have found it helpful to use a hash mark system; recording a mark in the margin of the paper for each new, significant, relative statement. Thus, the number of hash marks, compared to the established key, gives an objective indication of the adequacy of the discussion.

The essay, or discussion, test is an important instrument for use in the evaluation procedure. In addition to eliciting a response that can be compared to a standard, it provides the side benefits of developing one's abilities of expression and logical thinking. The essay test is also thought to be more effective in eliciting a future concern for the material being tested. Whereas upon completing a short answer test there is a tendency to feel that "that is it," with the essay test there is greater likelihood that the person may think of more that might have been said. Thus the essay test may have greater carryover value. Furthermore, the person who is prepared for the essay test will also be prepared for the short answer test.

administration procedures

When the test items have been constructed, the directions for taking the test should be developed, a scoring key prepared, and other details arranged. The test is then ready for trial application and subsequent refinement.

Use of Teacher Made Tests

Perhaps it should be pointed out that the teacher-made test for class use will have its so-called trial application in the first actual use with the class. Subsequent revisions and uses tend to give the teacher-made test some of the desirable qualities of the standardized test plus the desired specificity in relation to expected outcomes. In general, the good teacher-made test is superior to the standardized test for all purposes except for comparison of different groups.

One of the most serious abuses of the test is that its use is generally confined to determining marks. In addition to its use in the evaluation process, which includes much more than determining marks, the test can be one of the most effective teaching devices. Since it may be used to encourage self-evaluation, its use as a teaching device is, in reality, a part of the evaluation process. This is a far cry from simply testing to determine marks.

In addition to the direct benefits from varied use of tests, there is that of developing an acceptance of the test as contrasted with the common rejection of it when its use is confined to marking. The popularity of tests in newspapers and magazines indicates that people like to test themselves and to be tested. Tests are not liked because of the penalty attached to failure. Without reducing its effectiveness in the evaluation process, wide use of tests in other ways would serve to restore it to a place of respect.

In selecting the various evaluation procedures to be listed in the instructional unit plan, it should be kept in mind that tests and other evaluation procedures to be used for instructional purposes should be listed in the column with other methods, devices, and techniques. It is appropriate to list a suggested procedure or instrument both as a method, device, and technique and as an evaluation procedure, but the listing of a procedure in one place only serves to indicate its possible use in that connection and not in any other.

Knowledge outcomes may be evaluated through the use of test data. For this purpose a variety of kinds of tests and test items may be employed, including the traditional recitation. It is important to adjust the kind of item to the material being tested. In spite of the problem of objectivity of scoring, the essay test does have a prominent place in the procedure intended to evaluate health knowledge.

Attitude outcomes are difficult to evaluate. However, when viewed in their proper relationship to behavior it is apparent that observation of behavior (including anecdotal records) with objective recording of observations, will give a fair indication of attitudes. Attitude scales are valuable in self-evaluation, in counseling, and in group diagnosis. They are not valid for use in determining academic marks. Group diagnosis enables the instructor to determine areas of strength and weakness of the whole class and thus to adjust instruction to the needs of the pupils. The essay test provides a very effective means of observing attitudes as they may be elicited by a well-formulated question. Expressed student feelings and opinions also provide a partial basis for evaluating the success in attaining the expected outcomes.

Practice outcomes may be evaluated through observation, records, and practice inventories. Observations must be objective with an objective record. Health records, which cover, for example, immunizations, dental work, and illnesses, provide evidence of the effectiveness of instruction and thus become effective in providing data for use in the evaluation process. Practice inventories, like attitude scales, make their greatest contribution in the areas of self-evaluation and counseling. They are not valid for use in determining academic marks.

In developing the list of procedures to be used in evaluating the expected outcomes, it is important to remember that they are aimed at expected outcomes. There is no need for again listing what is to be evaluated since it appears in the expected outcomes section of the unit.

Need for Test Refinement

It is generally recognized that first attempts to construct good tests are often disappointing. In spite of all precautions, such defects as ambiguity, vocabulary burden, nondiscrimination (too easy or too hard), negative discrimination, lack of specificity, and imbalance tend to appear upon the first applications of the test. This fact has served to impress testors of the need for refining any test that may be used in more than one application. One of the chief characteristics of standardized tests, produced commercially, is that they are more highly refined than the common teacher-made tests. In many instances, this is about the only advantage such a test might have over the teacher-made test since the latter can be aimed more specifically at the outcomes desired in that particular situation. Another advantage of the teacher-made test is that it might include better balance for the intended use as well as greater specificity concerning the subject matter.

It is agreed that the teacher will not ordinarily use a test repeatedly, yet at the same time we must recognize that the important outcomes in a course do not change radically from semester to semester. In view of this, the construction of a test for a particular course or purpose becomes, in reality, a matter of improving upon previous tests. To this extent *much test construction becomes test refinement.*

For purposes of this discussion, it is assumed that steps one to four have been carried out, as discussed earlier in this chapter and that we have what appears to be a good test (face validity). Consideration is now given to the process of refining or improving the test, steps 5, 6, and 7 (see page 238).

The need for test refinement is ordinarily considered to be limited to developing the standardized test. However, this should not be the case. It is also a very important procedure for teachers who must test over the same material from year to year. To avoid using the same test items repeatedly, a large number of items may be developed from which the test items may be selected for any particular use. Since the items will be used in subsequent years, or for other sections of the same course, it is important that they be refined.

Refining the Health Education Test

At least six steps are customary in refining the health education test. These are (1) trial application (step 5), (2) statistical treatment for measures of central tendency and of distribution, (3) determination of a reliability coefficient, (4) item analysis, (5) elimination or revision of items (step 6), and (6) establishment of norms (step 7).

trial application

The trial application should provide enough cases to allow for an adequate sampling of students. Furthermore, the tests should contain many more items than needed in the refined test (probably twice the number). It is important to remember that the purpose of the trial application is to *test the test, not the student*. For a standardized test it has been variously estimated that 300 to 500 cases give an adequate number for refining the test. This number, of course, depends on the use to be made of the test. If it is to be used locally, fewer cases will give an adequate sampling of the population to be tested; a greater sampling will be needed for a test that is to be used on a wider scale. Enough subjects should be included to provide a representative sample of the group to be tested.

Since the ultimate purpose of refining the test is to produce a better test, the trial application of the test can provide data that may be used to improve the difficulty, improve the reliability, improve the validity and, if desired, provide equivalent forms of the test.

To make the results of the trial application useful, the trial application should possess these characteristics: (1) The group tested should resemble the group for which the test was made; (2) the group should have varying abilities, ideally following a normal distribution for a group of the kind for which the test was made; (3) everyone should complete the test; and (4) the test should be administered under controlled conditions.

central tendency and distribution

Statistical treatment of the data may include determining the simple measures of central tendency (mean, median, and mode) and of distribution (range and standard deviation). (6) The use of these data will be determined, in part, by the method of determining the reliability. However, in themselves, these data may be used to give some idea of the difficulty of the test and of the distribution of scores. If a number of items are removed from the test, the resulting test may have a lower reliability coefficient than the original test, even though it may be a better test. (1:156–157)

the reliability coefficient

The reliability coefficient *(r)* of the test may be determined in several ways. A simple and satisfactory method, involving only the use of statistics that are readily available, is a simplified form of the Kuder-Richardson formula below. This formula was developed by the simple procedure of carrying out the indicated operations in the Kuder-Richardson formula (1:154) and then further reducing the fraction to the form presented here.

$$r = \frac{N - \dfrac{M(N-M)}{\sigma^2}}{N-1}$$

where   r = reliability coefficent
σ = standard deviation
N = number of items in the test
M = mean of the test scores

It is worthy of note that the above formula may ordinarily be expected to give a conservative coefficient of reliability, if not an underestimate.

A second method of determining the reliability coefficient of the test may be by the use of the Pearson r; this involves the correlation of either (1) chance halves of the test, (2) equivalent forms of the test, or (3) repeated applications of the test (test, retest). If the chance halves method is selected, a more accurate estimate of the reliability of the whole test is secured through the application of the Spearman-Brown prophecy formula: (1:151)

$$r = \frac{2r_{12}}{1 + r_{12}}$$

where r = the reliability coefficient of the total test
r_{12} = the correlation between the scores on the halves of the test as represented by the Pearson r

Other things being equal, the longer the test the greater the reliability. A reliability coefficient of .90 or better is highly desirable if the test is to have more than local use.

item analysis

Item analysis involves two distinct approaches. The commonly accepted statistical approach must be supplemented by the logical approach. The teacher-made test for local use may well be subjected to intense study. The logical approach may be the more fruitful, particularly if the number of cases in the trial application has been limited. Furthermore, through introspection it may often be possible to improve an important though seemingly poor item and thus make it worthy of retention in the refined test. Any such revised items should be further subjected to trial application before appearing in a so-called refined test.

The statistical approach to item analysis involves identifying items that are not considered good items, the principal criterion in this instance being the discriminatory power of an item. A nondiscriminating item serves no purpose in the test intended for use as a basis for marking. Items, which are passed by everyone or failed by everyone, are immediately identified as nondiscriminating items. An item that is failed by more than 90 percent of the testees is too difficult and one that is failed by fewer than 10 percent is too easy. This figure will be determined, in part, by the use to be made of the test.

The difficulty of an item is expressed in terms of the proportion, or percentage, passing the item. When thus expressed, the more difficult item is expressed by a smaller proportion, or percentage. For example, an item passed by 10 percent of the group is more difficult than an item passed by 20 percent; hence the most difficult item has a difficulty level of zero, while the least difficult item has a difficulty level of 100.

Items that are failed as often by good students as by poor students or passed as often by poor students as by good students are considered poor items, since they fail to discriminate between the good and poor students. Similarly, items that are passed more frequently by poor students than by good ones discriminate adversely or negatively. Poor and negative discriminating items should either be revised and subjected to a second trial application or eliminated from the test if it is to be used for discriminating purposes.

To isolate the valid items, as determined by comparing the proportion of the upper group and the proportion of the lower group passing an item, it is acceptable to compare the approximately upper 27 percent of the students with the lower 27 percent. For the purpose of most tests, the difference between the proportion in the upper group who pass an item and the proportion in the lower group who pass the same item, should be at least three times the probable error (at the 5 percent level of confidence).

There are a number of procedures for identifying valid test items. Votaw (14:682–686) describes a graphical means of determining valid items. Flanagan (12:125–130) proposed an index of item validity, the Flanagan Index, which is easy to use and generally available in educational circles. Current computer programs for scoring tests usually provide these statistical data.

Even after the valid items have been identified by the statistical method, there often remains much that can be done to improve a test. There are at least two considerations regarding distractor functions: (1) Are all of the options being used? (2) Is the correct option being selected by good students more often than any of the distractors? Introspection plays a prominent role at this point, particularly if some of the options are not being selected.

eliminate or revise items

The logical approach, or refining the test through introspection, implies the necessity of discovering facts that are not revealed through statistical treatment. The necessity for revision of an option that is not functioning is an example of such an imperfection. Other qualities that may be revealed by critical examination of the items may be ambiguity, grammatical correctness, simplicity of statement, specificity of subject matter being tested, specific determiners, distractors that are not plausible, duplication, appearance of validity (face validity), curricular validity, and controversial items.

Final selection of the valid items to be used will depend upon several factors. It is essential to retain the balance of the test. Consequently, to sample some areas adequately, it may be necessary to use items that are not considered as good as other items in other areas. For example, in the health knowledge test, if a particular area such as nutrition has been assigned 8 percent of the emphasis, while another area such as relaxation has been assigned 4 percent, it may be more difficult to get 8 percent of good items in nutrition than it is to get 4 percent of good items in relaxation. Consequently, it may be necessary to retain some items in one area that are not as good as some items that must be discarded in the other areas.

The desired difficulty of the test will depend on the intended use of the test. Generally speaking, if the test is to be used to rank a group from high to low, the distribution of the items by difficulty should follow the general pattern of the so-called normal curve with an average difficulty of 50 percent. If the test is to screen out a few superior individuals, then the average difficulty should be greater than 50 percent; if it is to screen out a few inferior individuals the average difficulty should be less than 50 percent.

establish norms

The final step in refining the test is the establishing of norms. If the test is for local use only the test or a revision of it may be refined as it is administered from time to time. However, if the test is to have wide use, then it becomes desirable to establish norms for the entire area of usage. As with the trial application, the extent of usage will determine the number of cases necessary to establish satisfactory norms. The number of cases should vary approximately in proportion to the population to be tested. The greater the proportion of the population included in the norms, the better.

The reliability of the refined test may now be determined on the basis of the results of these applications of the test. As stated earlier, a reliability coefficient of .90 or better is highly desirable for a standardized test. A lower coefficient of reliability might be satisfactory for a teacher-made test for local classroom use.

Summary

Health educators must be aware that the appraisal of health education consists of much more than the use of the customary paper and pencil tests. They need to evaluate the total curriculum from the standpoint of the use of the curriculum guide by teachers and other school personnel, the success of predicting the achievements of the students, and the influence of the evaluation on subsequent planning.

Special consideration is given to the results of the instructional program in terms of attainment of the expected outcomes stated in the unit plans of the course of study and to the success of attaining the outcomes hoped for through the other aspects of the school health education program.

In view of the widespread use of health education tests, a great deal of commonsense must go into their construction and refinement. The original construction of the test is difficult, partly because of the controversial nature of much of the material and partly because our testing procedures and instruments make it extremely difficult to test many of the more desirable outcomes in this area. Statistical techniques are important in the process of refining the test, but let us not lose sight of the fact that *no amount of statistical treatment can create a truth out of a falsehood.*

In the last analysis, the quality of the health education test will be determined by: (1) The extent to which the test is in line with instructional objectives. (2) The adequacy of the sampling of the material being tested. (3) The specificity of the material being tested. (4) The quality of the individual items including validity, reliability, and objectivity. (5) The appropriateness of the vocabulary, that is, the vocabulary burden. (6) The appropriateness of the difficulty of the items. (7) The adequacy of directions and provisions for administering the test.

Finally, when the test is constructed and refined to meet these criteria, it must be used wisely if it is to serve the purpose for which it is constructed. It should be emphasized that testing is not an end in itself and that one of the many important purposes of testing is to furnish a partial basis for evaluation.

References

1. Adkins, D.C. et al., *Construction and Analysis of Achievement Tests,* U.S. Civil Service Commission, Washington, D.C., 1947

2. Anderson, C.L., *School Health Practice,* Fifth Edition, Mosby, St. Louis, 1972.

3. Barnhart, C.L., Editor, *The American College Dictionary,* Spencer, Chicago, 1948.

4. Beauchamp, G.A., *Curriculum Theory,* Third Edition, Kagg, Willmette, Illinois, 1975.

5. Goodlad, J.I., R. von Stoephasius, and M.F. Klein, *The Changing School Curriculum,* The Fund for the Advancement of Education, New York, 1966.

6 Lindquist, E.F., *A First Course in Statistics,* Houghton, Chicago, 1942.

7. Means, R.K., *Historical Perspectives on School Health,* Slack, Thorofare, N.J., 1975.

8. Patty, W.W., "Uses for Health Education Tests," *The Journal of School Health*, 19:3 (1949).

9. Pigg, R.M., Jr., *School Health Program Guidelines*, unpublished doctoral dissertation, Indiana University, Bloomington, 1974.

10. Pigg, R.M., Jr., "A History of School Health Program Evaluation in the United States," *The Journal of School Health*, 46:10 (1976).

11. Rash, J.K. et al., *School Health Program Evaluation, Tentative Standards and Score Sheet*, Department of Health and Safety Education, Indiana University, Bloomington, 1973.

12. Scott, M.G. and E. French, *Measurement and Evaluation in Physical Education*, Brown, Dubuque, Iowa, 1959.

13. Thordike, R.L., and E.P. Hagen, *Measurement and Evaluation in Psychology and Education*, Wiley, 1977.

14. Votaw, D.F., "Graphical Determination of Probable Error in Validation of Test Items," *Journal of Educational Psychology*, 24, December (1953).

15. Wilson, H.B., *An Instrument for Evaluating Health Instruction in Secondary Schools, Grades 9-12*, unpublished doctoral dissertation, Indiana University, Bloomington, 1960.

Chapter Twenty-One
The Past Is Prologue

In the three sections of this textbook we have dealt with three different aspects of health education curriculum development. Part I was concerned with health education curriculum foundations; Part II dealt with health education curriculum Design; and Part III was concerned with health education curriculum implementation and evaluation.

Health Education Curriculum Foundations

We have chosen to define the health education curriculum as *the systematic organization of courses, and of other activities, experiences, and situations that may favorably influence the health education development of the pupil.* By definition, then, the curriculum consists of *planned* experiences. Other experiences may make their contribution to education; but if they are to be considered as a part of the curriculum, they should be included in the written plans that we call the curriculum.

To paraphrase the words of a popular song, *whatever has been, has been.* In another vein, *our thoughts, unspoken, fall back dead, but no power can recall them once they are said.* The early history of health education is behind us and we cannot reenact the events that have transpired or correct the mistakes that have been made. However, we can point with pride to the fact that health education has come from an obscure beginning well within the lifetime of the senior members of the profession and has taken its place among the established professions. Today, it commands a position of respect, both in school health and public health, and health educators are recognized as essential members of the education team.

The progress made in the profession of health education is closely allied with the developing philosophies of health, education, and the role of education in health conservation. All of this has been in harmony with the emerging concept of the wholeness of the individual; the interdependence of the different aspects of life (physical, emotional, social, and spiritual); the recognition of the importance of early childhood experiences, and the realization that our lives are pretty much governed by our basic beliefs—our philosophy. As a result we now view health education as a lifetime process concerned primarily with helping each individual to intelligently direct his/her own health behavior to the end that health will be conserved.

We have proposed that health be defined as optimum physical, emotional, social, and spiritual well-being, and not merely the absence of disease or infirmity. This definition allows for different levels of health, with the goal for each individual being the optimum attainable level. The conservation of health will be concerned with health protection and promotion, correction of remedial defects, and adjusting to defects that cannot be corrected. Acceptance of the goal of intelligent self-direction of health behavior, as opposed to health as a goal, precludes undue emphasis on perfect health and the dangers that may result from making health the goal of life. You learn to do the best you can and live with the consequences.

In our society the school is recognized as the principal educational agency. This recognition often overlooks the tremendous educational impact of the home during early childhood and out of school life. Recognition of the influence of the home dictates that the success of the educational efforts depends to a great extent on the cooperative efforts of home and school personnel. Similarly, the nature of health education is such that many different disciplines of the school may make a significant impact on the health education of the students. In addition, success in health education depends to a considerable extent on involving different community personnel and programs in the total educational effort. The valuable assistance of the personnel of community health agencies is too often overlooked. In short, successful health education must be a cooperative effort of school, home, and community personnel.

Health Education Curriculum Design

The general principles of curriculum development have application in health education, but a few have special implications. The three step process of (1) general overview of the field of health education, (2) specific goal identification, and (3) revision of goals is particularly important in the rapidly changing field of health education. A second principle of special importance in health education curriculum development is to involve a large number and wide variety of individuals in

250

the planning process. This is important both from the point of view of the input of the individuals and of the possible education of the participants concerning the health education program. Other principles that have special application to health education include: the importance of example, the importance of early childhood experiences, the influence of an environment that is conducive to learning, and the principle of delayed response.

If the principle of wide participation is to be effective, special plans must be made for involving a large number of people in the planning process. Curriculum development is a constant three-step process: producing the curriculum, implementing the curriculum, and appraising the effectiveness of the curriculum and the curriculum process. The basic considerations in curriculum planning include administrative support, the curriculum project coordinator, the community wide health education curriculum advisory council, the health education curriculum committee, the central course of study committee, the instructional (or resource) unit committees, the tryout personnel and procedures, editing and publishing the course of study, and evaluating and revising the course of study. Each of these considerations leads logically to the next one, thus providing a smooth flow of responsibility from one step to the next. The entire process culminates in the revision of the course of study, which brings us back to step one. Thus, the continuous process of curriculum development is promoted.

According to our definition, the health education curriculum includes the planned educational experiences that may take place in several areas of the school outside of the health education classroom. These include the experiences in the health services, those in the environment (the healthful living experiences), and those in other classes. Such experiences are not limited to the school. The family physician, dentist, and pharmacist can be involved in the health education. Experiences can be planned that involve members of the police force, the fire department, the water and sanitation departments, and various other aspects of community services. The crucial and determining factor is the deliberate planning that is necessary to ensure that the student has those experiences and that they are educational. It is the responsibility of currciulum planners to see that this is accomplished.

Various patterns of scheduling and sequence of health instruction have been suggested. No attempt has been made to say that one pattern is superior to others. The crucial factor in each instance is that health education command the same consideration as any other discipline in the school program. Special emphasis should be placed on the importance of health education in helping establish desirable health attitudes and practices in the early grades and in providing assistance to the students in understanding and dealing with the health problems peculiar to their own situation.

The health education course of study comprises the heart of the health education curriculum. Although the other activities, experiences, and situations may make significant contributions; the health education class still provides the unique opportunity for bringing together varied experiences and for integrating them into a philosophy and a pattern of living that will truly conserve health in its broadest sense. Planning of the course of study should be a cooperative venture. While the major responsibility will rest with the teachers who will be using the course of study, others should be involved and consulted for their input. It is especially important that parents, students, and experts in the particular area (such as nutrition) be involved in the planning.

Just as the course of study constitutes the heart of the health education curriculum, so does the unit plan constitute the heart of the course of study. In spite of the varied approaches to planning for health education experiences, it is significant that they have so much in common. Almost all approaches provide for statements of objectives or pupil outcomes; content or subject matter to be used in achieving the expected outcomes; methods, devices, and techniques (or learning experiences); evaluation procedures; and references or sources of information to be used.

The importance of the stated expected outcomes is generally recognized. Considerable emphasis has been placed on how the expected outcomes are stated. In spite of the varied approaches in stating expected outcomes, there is general agreement that the student should be able to clearly perceive what behavior is expected. The statement of the expected outcomes provides the basis for planning the related health education experiences; hence, it must convey the message of what is expected of the learner. All content, methods, references, and evaluation procedures are selected with reference to their possible contribution to the realization of that particular outcome.

The opportunities for health education through healthful living and health service situations and experiences are often overlooked. If those opportunities are to be effective in the health education process, there must be conscious planning to take advantage of them. This calls for plans similar to the unit plans for the health education classes. These plans should be developed by representatives of the various departments concerned; for example, custodians, physicians, dentists, and nurses in cooperation with health educators, students, and parents. The environmental and health service staff members should be thoroughly familiar with those plans and should consult them from time to time in order to be more alert to the opportunities that may arise. These plans comprise an important part of the health education curriculum.

Health education through related subjects may be carried out either through correlated teaching, the integrated program, or incidental teaching. In any event a cooperatively developed unit plan, or a similar plan, should provide the guidelines for such instruction. It is important that these plans be coordinated with the plans for health instruction in all other aspects of the health education curriculum.

The methods, devices, and techniques to be used will depend on the nature of the subject matter selected for use in attaining the expected outcomes. They will also depend on the abilities and preferences of the instructor. In any event, a variety of methods, devices, and techniques should be suggested for each content item to provide an interesting variety of approaches and to allow for individual differences of students and instructors.

A philosophical approach to methodology leads to the conclusion that *the end is often inherent in the means.* In other words, the methods used in accomplishing a task determine the nature of the accomplishment. In health education, since the goal is *self-direction,* emphasis should be placed on such self-direction throughout the education process. The role of the instructor (for example, custodian, physician, dentist, nurse, and teacher) is to foster an environment that is conducive to learning. This can be accomplished in part by fostering a favorable physical and emotional climate, along with informing, interpreting, and inspiring as the opportunity arises.

Health Education Curriculum Implementation and Evaluation

If health education is to be successful, it must be a lifetime process. The importance of early experiences, of establishing desirable patterns of health behavior early in life, dictates that health education begin in the home. Furthermore, considering the long period after the school life of the individual and the constant and rapid changes in health knowledge, it is important that health education be continued throughout the lifetime of the individual. A number of community agencies share in the responsibility of providing preschool and post-school health education, and the school must share in that responsibility.

The school and the health department must carry the primary responsibility for lifetime health education. Other agencies, notably the voluntary health agencies, are willing and able to assist in the process. The cooperative efforts of all concerned can result in an effective health education program.

During the preschool years, the burden of education rests primarily with the home. The school can assist the parents by providing resource materials and opportunities for parent education classes, often in cooperation with the health department and voluntary agencies. The focus of this education will be the health education of the parents in order that they may provide a healthful environment and effective health education for their children during the preschool years.

The responsibilities of the school increase when the children enter school, but the parent responsibilities do not cease. Parents must continue to provide guidance to their children and thus support the efforts of the school. Parent involvement in school planning can significantly increase parent interest and support of the school program. Such involvement is important throughout the school life of the child. It is also important that students be involved in planning the health education curriculum.

In the selection of health problem areas, expected outcomes, and the accompanying educational materials and procedures, curriculum planners should be guided by the criteria of student and community needs, interests, comprehension abilities, community values, and the possibility of independent action by the students (dependency). When these criteria are used as guides in planning the health education curriculum, there is reasonable assurance that the program will be effective. There will be adequate consideration of student problems as they progress through their school life, with little danger of needless repetition or omission of important health problems. In secondary schools and colleges students should increasingly share the responsibilities associated with planning their own health education curriculum, and in the adult health education programs the students should have the major responsibility for such planning.

In the process of planning the secondary school, college, and adult health education programs there is danger that fleeting student interests may become the determining factor in selecting the problem areas. Important as interests are, they should not be the sole criterion, and this can be avoided if the recommended procedures and accepted critieria are recognized and followed in the planning process. Emphasis on health needs, and related health education needs, will preclude the exclusive use of interests as the criterion for determining the nature of the curriculum.

The college and university health education programs may be either voluntary (elective) or required, but the adult programs will be completely elective. The citizens will have complete freedom of choice to read health articles in newspapers and magazines, to listen to radio and television, to attend special lectures on community health problems, and to attend health education classes. As a result, the health education program for adults must be attractive. In a sense, educators are obligated to provide the citizens with programs they need and give them reason to like it. In fact, this should be the guiding principle throughout all of education. If more emphasis were placed on conducting the health education programs in such a way as "to make them like it," there would be fewer failures. Greater emphasis should be placed on fostering an environment that is conducive to learning.

In view of the nature of health education, evaluation is an even more important aspect of curriculum development than it is in some other disciplines. Not only is health information changing rapidly, but the instability of desirable health practices and the individual differences of students make it imperative that evaluation be a continuous, ongoing, process.

254

Evaluation may take different forms. In addition to health instruction, total program evaluation may include consideration of administrative provisions and procedures, environmental situations and practices, and health service programs. Even when limited to the health instruction program, evaluation should consider the contributions made to health education by other aspects of the school program, including all of the components of the health educaiton curriculum.

Total program evaluation is probably best accomplished by an evaluation team made up of selected representatives of the local school under the leadership of a person skilled in evaluation procedures. This person is often called an outside expert. This procedure has the advantage of the expertise of the expert while involving those who have a part in conducting the program and who will have the responsibility of carrying out the recommendations of the evaluators. The personal growth of those involved will be an added benefit, both to the individual and the school.

A variety of procedures may be used in appraising the results of the health instruction program. *Practice outcomes* may be evaluated by direct observation, practice inventories, student reports, parent observation and reports, and by observing and recording the health results of certain practices. For example, the overweight student may reduce by following the proper diet; the student can avoid certain communicable diseases by vaccination; and personal appearance can be influenced through well-known practices. *Attitude outcomes* are more difficult to evaluate, but attitude inventories are effective, provided there is no penalty attached to honest reporting. Teacher and parent observation of behavior, which is influenced by attitudes, is effective in many instances. Student reporting and discussion of personal attitudes serves both as a means of evaluating and a teaching procedure. *Knowledge outcomes* are the easiest to appraise. As a result, too much appraisal in health education is based on health knowledge tests with the result that the emphasis in teaching is often almost exclusively on health knowledge. Knowledge is important, especially in the upper grades and adult programs but, unless it is applied in practice, it is of little value for personal health. As a result, more and better ways of evaluating attitudes and practices must be devised. This is a never-ending challenge to health educators.

Since health education tests are in common use, and will continue to be used, the construction of such tests becomes one of the important responsibilities of the health educator. Special concern should be shown for constructing attitude scales and practice inventories that may be used for personal evaluation and counseling as well as group diagnosis. In the test used for group diagnosis the individual is rarely identified; thus it may be considered to be more valid than when the individual is identified, and the test may have the possibility of being used to determine academic marks.

Standardized tests have their place in pretesting to determine the needs and

255

accomplishments of students, but they are of limited use in evaluating the results of instruction in a given situation. The good teacher-made test is much more effective, since it can be focused on the particular concerns of the class. Health educators should be especially concerned that they develop the ability to construct good health education tests; attitude scales, practice inventories, and knowledge tests. However, testing should not preclude the use of other means of evaluating the health education curriculum.

Looking Ahead

The past is prologue. It is what is in the future that is most important. We have reached the point in health education as a profession where we now have, for the first time in the history of the profession, health educators who are receiving their undergraduate and graduate preparation in health education under the guidance of instructors who, themselves, had undergraduate and graduate preparation in health education. The early leaders in health education were persons of vision, often physicians, who had no special health education preparation but who saw the need for health education and took the lead in promoting it. Their students became the first generation of health educators, and now their students (YOU) have the opportunity to be the best prepared health educators in the history of the profession.

Innovation has become the name of the game, not only in health education but in education in general. New problems, new approaches, and new methods all add up to an exciting future for health educators. This is good, *but* it must be remembered that change is not necessarily progress. One of the principles of education is that progress comes slowly. Rejecting a new approach is as logical as accepting it.

It is difficult to evaluate success in health education in a short period of time. Some aspects of health education seem to be a two generation process. Even in instances where there is academic acceptance of health instruction, such as the dangers of smoking, the individual may not be able to subscribe fully to the practice. However, there is a much better possibility that the children (or students) of such a person will be able to accept fully the practice and, under the leadership of the enlightened parent and/or teacher, they may take one more step in the direction of intelligent self-direction of their health behavior.

While there is considerable merit in the concept that education is to prepare for adult living; the needs, opportunities, and contributions of the student as a citizen cannot be ignored. The student of any age is just as much a citizen as he or she will be at any other age. The responsibilities of the elementary school student, as a citizen, may differ considerably from those of the adult; but they are there, and the student should be encouraged to accept them and thus to contribute to life in the community. Furthermore, since every student is a citizen the converse is also true, and every citizen is (or should be) a student. This is especially true in relation to health and the solution of health problems. The health problem situation in the world is not static. Indeed, new diseases are constantly appearing and being identified. If the citizens are to intelligently direct their own health behavior they must keep abreast of new developments in the health field, this can only be accomplished through constant observation and study of new developments and by knowing where to go for counsel. Lifetime health education is essential if this is to be accomplished. This implies not only education for a lifetime but education throughout a lifetime.

If the school and community health education program (and it is one program) is to be effective, it must be planned effectively. In addition to the planning suggested for developing, implementing, and evaluating the curriculum, additional consideration should be given to the problems associated with coordination of the program. It is entirely possible that the most important action a school board could take to improve the health education program would be to appoint a *health coordinator* (Chapter 4). The health coordinator should be free to work cooperatively with all community health agency personnel to ensure a cooperative working relationship. Such a person would *not* need authority to direct action because it must be assumed that when the people know what action is desirable they will attempt to take that action. The coordinator must inspire the members of the staff, working as a motivator and a support agent to get the desirable action. The most effective approach of the coordinator is illustrated by the old Chinese saying, "the best leadership is that which, when the task is finished, the people will say, we did it ourselves."

In looking to the future, health education must be considered as a *psychological challenge*. It will not be too difficult to foster a favorable physical and emotional climate for the learner. Information will be readily available. Understanding of health problems, their prevention and solution, can be increased through explanation and interpretation. The crucial task of the health educator is to motivate or inspire the learner to put into his or her daily life the practices that are known to foster a high level of wellness. This action must be taken by the individual, personally. Parents, teachers, school administrators, health service personnel, members of the environmental health staff, public health officials, representatives of voluntary health agencies, and other professional health personnel can, and must, work together to foster an environment that is conducive to learning. The most important aspect of such an environment is the motivational or inspirational aspect, and the health educator is in a position to give leadership to such efforts.

Appendix A
Selected Sources of Information on Competency Based Education

The sources of information listed below provide interested health educators with a representative listing of sources from which general information concerning competency based education may be obtained. Individuals desiring information about the concept of competency based education are encouraged to contact the selected sources.

1. ERIC Clearinghouse on Teacher Education
   One Dupont Circle, NW
   Washington, D.C. 20036
2. PBTE Information Center
   American Association of Colleges for Teacher Education
   One Dupont Circle, Suite 610
   Washington, D.C. 20036
3. Teacher Education Center
   College of Education
   University of Georgia
   Athens, Georgia 30602
4. Pennsylvania Department of Education
   Box 911
   Harrisburg, Pennsylvania 17126
5. Texas Education Agency
   201 East 11th Street
   Austin, Texas 78701
6. Performance Evaluation Project
   New Jersey State Department of Education
   Trenton, New Jersey 08605

7. Office of Teacher Education and Certification
   New York State Department of Education
   Albany, New York 12201
8. National Commission on Performance Based Education
   Educational Testing Service
   Princeton, New Jersey 08540
9. American Alliance for Health, Physical Education, and Recreation
   1201 16th Street, NW
   Washington, D.C. 20036
10. Research and Development Center for Teacher Education
    The University of Texas
    Austin, Texas 78712
11. College of Education
    University of Houston
    Houston, Texas 77004
12. Stanford Center for Research and Development in Teaching
    Stanford University
    Stanford, California 94305
13. Consortium of Competency Based Education Centers
    P.O. Box 20011
    Tallahassee, Florida 32304
14. National Institute of Education
    1200 19th Street, NW
    Washington, D.C. 20208
15. Phi Delta Kappa
    Eighth and Union
    Bloomington, Indiana 47401
16. National Resource and Dissemination Center
    Division of Educational Resources
    University of South Florida
    Tampa, Florida 33620
17. National Council for Accreditation of Teacher Education
    1950 Pennsylvania Avenue, NW
    Washington, D.C. 20006
18. National Dissemination Center for Performance Based Education
    150 Marshall Street
    Syracuse University
    Syracuse, New York 13201

Competency Based Education References

"A Special Issue on Competency/Performance-Based Teacher Education," *Phi Delta Kappan*, 55:290–343 (January, 1974).

Houston, W.R., Editor, *Exploring Competency Based Education*, McCutchan, Berkeley, 1974.

Houston, W.R. and R.B. Howsam, Editors, *Competency Based Teacher Education: Progress, Problems, and Prospects*, Science Research Associates, Chicago, 1972.

Levy, M.R., W.H. Green, and F.H. Jenne, "Competency-Based Professional Preparation," *School Health Review* 3:4 (May–June, 1972).

Netcher, J.R., *A Management Model for Competency-Based HPER Programs*, Mosby, St. Louis, 1977.

Pigg, R.M., "A National Study of Competency Based Health Education Programs," *Health Education*, 7:15–16 (July–August, 1976)

Pigg, R.M., *Competency Based Health Education: An Overview*, Teacher Education Center, College of Education, University of Georgia, Athens, 1975.

Pigg, R.M., "Defining Competency Based Health Education," *Eta Sigma Gamman*, 7:16–17 (Autumn, 1975).

Shearron, G.F. and C.E. Johnson, *A CBTE Program in Action: University of Georgia*, Teacher Education Center, College of Education, University of Georgia, Athens, 1973.

Weigand, J.E., Editor, *Developing Teacher Competencies*, Prentice-Hall, Englewood Cliffs, N.J., 1971.

Selected Sources of Teaching Aids and References

Student Textbook Publishers: Elementary and/or Secondary Level

CEBCO Standard Publishing
104 Fifth Avenue
New York, New York 10011

Curriculum Innovations, Inc.
501 Lake Forest Avenue
Highwood, Illinois 60040

Globe Book Company, Inc.
175 Fifth Avenue
New York, New York 10010

Harcourt, Brace and Jovanovich
757 Third Avenue
New York, New York 10017

Holt, Rinehart, and Winston, Inc.
383 Madison Avenue
New York, New York 10017

Houghton Mifflin Company
One Beacon Street
Boston, Massachusetts 02107

Laidlaw Brothers
Thatcher and Madison
River Forest, Illinois 60305

J.P. Lippincott Company
East Washington Square
Philadelphia, Pennsylvania 19105

McGraw-Hill Book Company, Inc.
Princeton Road
Hightstown, New Jersey 08520

Scott, Foresman and Company
1900 East Lake Avenue
Glenview, Illinois 60025

Student Textbook Publishers: College Level

Allyn and Bacon, Inc.
470 Atlantic Avenue
Boston, Massachusetts 02210

Lea and Febiger
600 S. Washington Square
Philadelphia, Pennsylvania 19106

C.V. Mosby Company
3301 Washington Blvd.
St. Louis, Missouri 63103

D. Van Nostrand Company
450 West 33rd Street
New York, New York 10001

Harper and Row, Inc.
49 East 33rd Street
New York, New York 10016

Holt, Rinehart, and Winston, Inc.
383 Madison Avenue
New York, New York 10017

Houghton Mifflin Company
One Beacon Street
Boston, Massachusetts 02107

John Wiley & Sons, Inc.
605 Third Avenue
New York, New York 10016

Macmillan Publishing Company
866 Third Avenue
New York, New York 10022

Mayfield Publishing Company
285 Hamilton Avenue
Palo Alto, California 94301

McGraw-Hill Book Company
Princeton Road
Hightstown, New Jersey 08520

Prentice Hall, Inc.
Englewood Cliffs, New Jersey 07632

Random House
201 E. 50th Street
New York, New York 10022

W.B. Saunders Company
W. Washington Square
Philadelphia, Pennsylvania 19105

William C. Brown Publishers
135 S. Locust Street
Dubuque, Iowa 52001

Teacher References: Methodology in Health Education

Barrett, M., *Health Education Guide*, Second Edition, Lea and Febiger, Philadelphia, 1974.

Bruess, C.E. and J.E. Gay, *Implementing Comprehensive School Health*, Macmillan, New York, 1978.

Cornacchia, H.J., D.E. Smith, and D.J. Bental, *Drugs in the Classroom*, Second Edition, Mosby, St. Louis, 1978.

Cornacchia, H.J. and W.M. Staton, *Health in Elementary Schools*, Mosby, St. Louis, 1974.

Engs, R.C., S.E. Barnes, and M. Wantz, *Health Games Students Play*, Fourth Edition, Mosby, St. Louis, 1974.

Engs, R. and M. Wantz, *Teaching Health Education in the Elementary School*, Houghton Mifflin, Boston, 1978.

Ensor, P.G. and R.K. Means, *Instructor's Resource and Methods Handbook for Health Education*, Second Edition, Allyn and Bacon, Boston, 1977.

Fodor, J.T. and G.T. Dalis, *Health Instruction: Theory and Application*, Second Edition, Lea and Febiger, Philadelphia, 1974.

Galli, N., *Foundations and Principles of Health Education*, Wiley, New York, 1978.

Greenberg, J.S., *Student-Centered Health Instruction: A Humanistic Approach*, Addison-Wesley, Reading, Massachusetts, 1978.

Greene, W.H., F.H. Jenne, and P.M. Legos, *Health Education in the Elementary School*, Macmillan, New York, 1978.

Grout, Ruth E., *Health Teaching in Schools*, Saunders, Philadelphia, 1968.

Haag, J.H., *School Health Program*, Third Edition, Lea & Febiger, Philadelphia, 1972.

Humphrey, J.H., W.R. Johnson, and D.R. Nowack, *Health Teaching in Elementary Schools*, Thomas, Springfield, Illinois, 1975.

Jenne, F.H. and W.H. Greene, *Turner's School Health and Health Education*, Mosby, St. Louis, 1976.

Kime, R.E., R.G. Schlaadt, and L.E. Tritsch, *Health Instruction: An Action Approach*, Prentice-Hall, Englewood Cliffs, New Jersey, 1977.

Mayshark, C. and R.A. Foster, *Health Education in Secondary Schools*, Third Edition, Mosby, St. Louis, 1972.

Mayshark, C. and R.A. Foster, *Methods in Health Education*, Mosby, St. Louis, 1966.

Nemir, A. and W.E. Schaller, *The School Health Program*, Saunders, Philadelphia, 1975.

Oberteuffer, D., O.A. Harrellson, and M.B. Pollock, *School Health Education*, Harper and Row, New York, 1972.

Read, D.A., *Looking In: Exploring One's Personal Health Values*, Prentice-Hall, Englewood Cliffs, New Jersey, 1977.

Read, D.A. and W.H. Greene, *Creative Teaching in Health*, Macmillan, New York, 1975.

Read, D.A., S.B. Simon, and J.B. Goodman, *Health Education: The Search for Values*, Prentice-Hall, Englewood Cliffs, New Jersey, 1977.

Russell, R.D., *Health Education*, National Education Association, Washington, D.C., 1975.

Savitz, B., Editor, *Go To Health*, Dell, New York, 1972.

Schneider, R.E., *Methods and Materials of Health Education*, Second Edition, Saunders, Philadelphia, 1964.

Somers, A.R., *Health Promotion and Consumer Health Education*, Prodist, New York, 1976.

Sorochan, W.D., *Personal Health Appraisal*, Wiley, New York, 1976.

Sorochan, W.D. and S.J. Bender, *Teaching Elementary Health Science*, Addison-Wesley, Reading Massachusetts, 1975.

Sorochan, W.D. and S.J. Bender, *Teaching Secondary Health Science*, Wiley, New York, 1978.

Vannier, M., *Teaching Health in Elementary Schools*, Second Edition, Lea and Febiger, Philadelphia, 1974.

Willgoose, C.E., *Health Education in the Elementary School*, Fourth Edition, Saunders, Philadelphia, 1974.

Willgoose, C.E., *Health Teaching in Secondary Schools*, Second Edition, Saunders, Philadelphia, 1977.

Selected Health Education Tests

Elementary Level

AAHPER Cooperative Health
  Education Test
Preliminary Form A
Educational Testing Service
Princeton, New Jersey 08540

Health Behavior Inventory
  (Elementary)
California Test Bureau
Del Monte Research Park
Monterey, California 93940

Junior High/Middle School Level

AAHPER Cooperative Health
  Education Test
Form 3A
Educational Testing Service
Princeton, New Jersey 08540

Health Behavior Inventory (Junior
  High)
California Test Bureau
Del Monte Research Park
Monterey, California 93940

Senior High School Level

Health Behavior Inventory
  (Senior High)
California Test Bureau
Del Monte Research Park
Monterey, California 93940

Fast-Tyson Health Knowledge Test
Department of Health and Physical
  Education
Northeast Missouri State University
Kirksville, Missouri 63501

College Level

Health Behavior Inventory (College)
California Test Bureau
Del Monte Research Park
Monterey, California 93940

Madison Health Knowledge Test
Department of Health and Physical
  Education
James Madison University
Harrisonburg, Virginia 22801

Kilander-Leach Health Knowledge Test
116 North Pleasant Avenue
Ridgewood, New Jersey 07450

Periodicals

Accident Facts
National Safety Council
444 N. Michigan Avenue
Chicago, Illinois 60611

American Journal of Public Health
American Public Health Association
1015 Eighteenth Street, NW
Washington, D.C. 20036

Consumer Reports
Consumer's Union, Inc.
Mount Vernon, New York 10850

Eta Sigma Gamman
Eta Sigma Gamma
2000 University Avenue
Muncie, Indiana 47306

Family Health (and *Today's Health*)
Family Health Magazine
Portland Place
Boulder, Colorado 80302

Health Bulletin for Teachers
Metropolitan Life Insurance
   Company
One Madison Avenue
New York, New York 10010

Health Education
Association for the Advancement of
   Health Education
1202 16th Street, NW
Washington, D.C. 20036

*International Journal of Health
Education*
International Union of Health
   Education
3 rue Viollier
Geneva, Switzerland

*Journal of the American College
Health Association*
American College Health
   Association
2807 Central Street
Evanston, Illinois 60201

Journal of School Health, The
American School Health Association
P.O. Box 708
Kent, Ohio 44240

Science Digest
Science Digest, Inc.
P.O. Box 10076
Des Moines, Iowa 50340

Voluntary and Professional Sources

Action for Children's Television
46 Austin Street
Newtonville, Massachusetts 02160

Action on Smoking and Health
P.O. Box 19556
Washington, D.C. 20006

Alcoholics Anonymous
P.O. Box 459
Grand Central Annex
New York, New York 10017

American Cancer Society
777 Third Avenue
New York, New York 10017

American Dental Association
211 E. Chicago Avenue
Chicago, Illinois 60611

American Dietetic Association
430 N. Michigan Avenue
Chicago, Illinois 60611

American Heart Association
44 E. 23rd Street
New York, New York 10010

American Hospital Association
840 N. Lake Shore Drive
Chicago, Illinois 60611

American Lung Association
1740 Broadway
New York, New York 10019

American Medical Association
535 N. Dearborn Street
Chicago, Illinois 60610

American National Red Cross
17th and D Streets, NW
Washington, D.C. 20006

American School Health Association
P.O . Box 708
Kent, Ohio 44240

American Social Health Association
173 Walton St., NW
Atlanta, Georgia 30303

Association for the Advancement of
Health Education
1201 16th Street, NW
Washington, D.C. 20036

National Center for Health
Education
44 Montgomery Street, Suite 2564
San Francisco, California 94104

National Safety Council
444 N. Michigan Avenue
Chicago, Illinois 60611

National Science Teachers
Association
1742 Connecticut Avenue, NW
Washington, D.C. 20009

Nutrition Foundation, Inc.
888 17th St., NW
Washington, D.C. 20006

Public Affairs Committee
381 Park Avenue South
New York, New York 10016

Commercial and Sponsored Sources

A.J. Nystrom and Company
3333 Elston Avenue
Chicago, Illinois 60618

American Bakers Association
1700 Pennsylvania Avenue, NW
Washington, D.C. 20006

American Institute of Baking
400 E. Ontario Street
Chicago, Illinois 60611

American Automobile Association
1712 G Street, NW
Washington, D.C. 22036

Cereal Institute, Inc.
1111 Plaza Drive
Schaumburg, Illinois 60195

Channing L. Bete Company, Inc.
45 Federal Street
Greenfield, Maryland 01301

Cleveland Health Museum
8911 Euclid Avenue
Cleveland, Ohio 44106

Colgate Palmolive Company
740 N. Rush Street
Chicago, Illinois 60611

Denoyer-Geppert
5235 Ravenswood Avenue
Chicago, Illinois 60640

Distilled Spirits Council of the U.S.,
Inc.
1300 Pennsylvania Building
Washington, D.C. 20004

Eli Lilly Company
740 S. Alabama Street
Indianapolis, Indiana 46206

General Mills, Inc.
P.O. Box 1113
Minneapolis, Minnesota 55420

Hubbard
P.O. Box 105
Northbrook, Illinois 60062

Johnson and Johnson
501 George Street
New Brunswick, New Jersey 08903

Kemper Insurance Companies
110 Tenth Avenue
Fulton, Illinois 61252

Kimberly-Clark Corporation
6701 W. Oakton
Chicago, Illinois 60648

Lederle Laboratories
Public Relations Department
Pearl River, New York 10965

Medical Plastics Laboratory
P.O. Box 38
Gatesville, Texas 76528

Metropolitan Life Insurance
1 Madison Avenue
New York, New York 10010

National Dairy Council
6300 N. River Rd.
Rosemont, Illinois 60018

National Nutrition Education
Clearinghouse
P.O. Box 931
Berkeley, California 94701

Personal Products Company
Consumer Information Center
Milltown, New Jersey 08850

Pharmaceutical Manufacturer's
Association
1155 15th Street, NW
Washington, D.C. 20005

Proctor and Gamble Company
Public Relations, Gwynne Building
Cincinnati, Ohio 45201

Public Relations Manager
McDonald's Corporation
One McDonald Plaza
Oak Brook, Illinois 60521

Hach Chemical Company
P.O. Box 907
Ames, Iowa 50010

School Health Supply Company
300 Lombard Road
Addison, Illinois 60101

Science Research Associates, Inc.
259 E. Erie Street *
Chicago, Illinois 60611

Spenco Medical Corporation
P.O. Box 8113
Waco, Texas 76710

Tampax, Inc.
P.O. Box 271
Palmer, Maryland 01069

Trend Enterprises, Inc.
P.O. Box 3073
St. Paul, Minnesota 55165

269

Audio-Visual Sources

Aims Instructional Media Services, Inc.
P.O. Box 1010
Hollywood, California 90028

Audio Visual Center
Indiana University
Bloomington, Indiana 47401

BFA Educational Media
2211 Michigan Avenue
Santa Monica, California 90404

Churchill Films
662 N. Robertson Blvd.
Los Angeles, California 90069

DCA Educational Products, Inc.
4865 Stenton Avenue
Philadelphia, Pennsylvania 19144

Educational Activities, Inc.
P.O. Box 392
Freeport, New York 11520

Guidance Associates
757 Third Avenue
New York, New York 10017

Marshfilm Enterprises, Inc.
P.O. Box 8082
Shawnee Mission, Kansas 66208

Modern Talking Picture Services, Inc.
2323 New Hyde Park Road
New Hyde Park, New York 11040

National Medical Audiovisual
   Center (Annex)
Center for Disease Control
Atlanta, Georgia 30333

Parents Magazine Films, Inc.
52 Vanderbilt Avenue
New York, New York 10017

Perennial Education, Inc.
P.O. Box 855, Ravinia
Highland Park, Illinois 60035

Pyramid Films
Box 1048
Santa Monica, California 90406

Sunburst Communications
39 Washington Avenue
Pleasantville, New York 01570

Walt Disney Educational Media
500 S. Buena Vista Street
Burbank, California 91521

Government Sources

Bureau of Community Health
   Services
Health Services Administration
U.S. Department of HEW
Washington, D.C. 20201

Bureau of Health Education
Center for Disease Control
Atlanta, Georgia 30333

Bureau of Product Safety
5401 Westbard Avenue
Bethesda, Maryland 20016

Consumer Product Information
Superintendent of Documents
Pueblo, Colorado 81009

Drug Enforcement Administration
U.S. Department of Justice
1405 I Street, NW
Washington, D.C. 20537

Environmental Protection Agency
Forms and Publications Center
Research Triangle Park, North
   Carolina 27711

Federal Trade Commission
6th Street and Pennsylvania Avenue,
   NW
Washington, D.C. 20580

Food and Drug Administration
Office of Public Affairs
Rockville, Maryland 20857

U.S. Department of Agriculture
Office of Communication
Washington, D.C. 20250

Inquiries Branch
Public Health Service
U.S. Department of HEW
Washington, D.C. 20025

National Highway Traffic Safety
   Administration
U.S. Department of Transportation
Washington, D.C. 20590

National Clearinghouse for Alcohol
   Information
P.O. Box 2345
Rockville, Maryland 20852

National Institute on Drug Abuse
11400 Rockville Pike
Rockville, Maryland 20852

National Institute of Mental Health
5600 Fishers Lane
Rockville, Maryland 20852

National Institute for Occupational
   Safety and Health
Center for Disease Control
Atlanta, Georgia 30333

National Interagency Council on
   Smoking and Health
Center for Disease Control
Atlanta, Georgia 30333

Office of Child Development
U.S. Department of HEW
Washington, D.C. 20013

Office of Public Affairs
Alcohol, Drug Abuse, and Mental
   Health Administration
5600 Fishers Lane
Rockville, Maryland 20852

Product Safety Information Division
U.S. Consumer Product Safety
   Commission
Washington, D.C. 20207

Public Inquiries and Report Branch
National Institutes of Health
Bethesda, Maryland 20014

271

Appendix C
Sample Units

Throughout the book, emphasis is placed on the importance of following a definite procedure in planning units of instruction in health education. To illustrate the planning process, 10 sample units have been prepared based on the procedures suggested in the book. The sample units should not be confused with complete teaching units. Their pupose is to illustrate the planning process rather than to provide complete teaching materials. A variety of additional expected outcomes and related content would need to be added to convert the sample units to teaching units.

Sample units have been prepared on various topics for kindergarten through older adulthood. The health problem area, title, long range goal, and expected outcomes have been designated for each unit. Selected content or subject matter has been included to illustrate the type of factual information that would contribute to the achievement of the outcomes. Methods, teaching aids, procedures for evaluation, and selected teacher and student references are listed for each unit.

The sample unit for grades K-1, *Traveling Safely To And From School*, is presented in the horizontal format suggested in Figure 8 of the text. The remaining sample units are presented in the vertical outline format, since the vertical format is often easier to prepare. However, unit planning procedures are the same regardless of the format utilized. In either case an expected outcome is identified, appropriate content or subject matter is selected, teaching aids are specified, and evaluation procedures are planned. When the plan for accomplishing the first expected outcome is completed, the same procedure is applied to the next outcome. When the vertical format is utilized, care should be taken to show the relationship between the expected outcome and the related content by using standard outline format procedures.

Problem Area: *Safety*

Title: *TRAVELING SAFELY TO AND FROM SCHOOL*

Long Range Goal: *Leads an active, vigorous life free from preventable accidents.*

Grade: *K-1*

Expected Outcomes	Content	Methods, Devices and Techniques	Teaching Aids	Evaluation Procedures	References: Teacher, Student
The student: 1. Understands that dangers may exist in traveling to and from school.	1. A. Hazards may exist when riding a bus or bicycle or when walking. B. Animals should not be bothered. C. Strangers should be avoided.	Resource speaker (policeman, safety patrol officer, etc.) Survey how children get to and from school. Role play proper car and bus conduct.	Street map Transportation safety posters Role-playing props	Questioning Observation Parent checklist	*Teacher:* As You Grow, Teacher's Ed., Harcourt, Brace, Jovanovich, New York, 1977. Fodor, J.T. et al., *Your Health,* Teacher Edition, Laidlaw, River Forest, Illinois, 1974. Richmond, J.B., et al. *You and Your Health,* Blue Level Teacher's Edition, Scott Foresman, Glenview, Illinois, 1977.
2. Examines the possibility that injury or death may result from unsafe practices or unsafe conditions.	2. A. Obey all traffic regulations. B. Weather factors affect safety. C. Bicycle safety rules should be followed. D. Bus courtesy may prevent accidents.	Diagram best route to school. Conduct field trip to observe intersections Practice safe street crossing. Practice meeting strangers.			Sorochan, W.D., and S.J. Bender, *Teaching Elementary Health Science,* Addison-Wesley, Reading, Massachusetts, 1975. Worick, W.W., *Safety Education,* Prentice-Hall, Englewood Cliffs, New Jersey, 1975.
3. Realizes individual attitude is important to safety.	3. A. Positive safety attitudes are helpful. B. Negative safety attitudes are harmful. C. Good passengers promote safety. D. The policeman is a friend.				*Student:* Greene, C., *What Do They Do, Policemen and Firemen?,* Harper and Row, New York, 1962. Kessler, L., *A Tale of Two Bicycles: Safety on Your Bike,* Lothrop, Lee and Shepard, New York, 1971.
4. Locates the safest route to and from school.	4. A. On route to school, knows location of: traffic controls, crosswalks, intersections, special hazards. B. Obey safety patrol.				McDonald, G., *Red Light, Green Light,* Doubleday, Garden City, New York, 1973. Shapp, M., and C. Shapp, *Let's Find Out About Safety,* Watts, New York, 1975.

Problem Area: *Nutrition*   Grade: *3*

Title: *GROWING AND EATING*

Long Range Goal: *Selects and eats a well balanced diet.*

Expected Outcomes
The student:
1. understands that proper nutrition is essential for growth.
2. identifies foods from each of the four food groups.
3. accepts the attitude that proper nutrition is important.
4. selects and eats foods from the four food groups.
5. prepares simple and nutritious snacks.
6. exhibits proper table manners while eating.

Content
*1. A.   All living organisms require food to grow.
     B.   Energy for bodily processes comes from food.
     C.   Food assists in body growth and repair.
     D.   Physical appearance is enhanced by proper nutrition.
 2. A.   The four food groups include:
          (1) meat group.
          (2) fruit and vegetable group.
          (3) milk group.
          (4) bread and cereal group.
     B.   Each of the four groups meet specific nutritional needs of the body.
     C.   Major nutrients include vitamins, minerals, fats, carbohydrates, protein, water, and fiber.
 3. A.   Proper nutrition helps prevent a number of diseases.
     B.   Personal growth and development depends on adequate nutrition.
     C.   Breakfast is an important factor in an enjoyable morning.
 4. A.   Selecting the proper number of servings from each group is essential to a balanced diet.
     B.   Selecting a variety of foods promotes a balanced diet.
 5. A.   Snacks may be nutritious or nonnutritious.
     B.   Several types of nutritious snacks are available.
     C.   Nutritious snacks are easy to prepare.
 6. A.   Eating utensils should be arranged neatly on the table.
     B.   The atmosphere should be relaxed and pleasurable while eating.
     C.   Do not speak while chewing.

* numbers refer to expected outcomes.

Methods
Demonstrate the effect of fertilizer on the growth of plants.
Conduct various dietary experiments using animals.
View pictures of healthy, happy, well-nourished children.
Construct food group posters or mobiles from magazine pictures.

Keep a food consumption record for several days.
Prepare several simple, nutritious snacks at school.
Set a table properly.
Practice using proper manners while dining.
View films or filmstrips concerning nutrition.

Aids
Plants or seeds
Fertilizer
Laboratory animals
Magazines
Cookbooks or recipes
Food for snacks
Kitchen utensils
Table settings
Film or filmstrip

Evaluation
Test observation
Project evaluation
Nutrition practice inventory

References
Teacher:
You Make Choices, Teacher's Edition, Harcourt, Brace & Jovanovich, New York, 1977.
Fodor, J.T. et al., *Your Health and You*, Teacher's Edition, Laidlaw, River Forest, Illinois, 1974.
Richmond, J.B. et al., *You and Your Health*, Red Level Teacher's Edition, Scott Foresman, Glenview, Illinois, 1977.
Sorochan, W.D. and S.J. Bender, *Teaching Elementary Health Science*, Addison-Wesley, Reading, Massachusetts, 1975.
White, P.L., *Let's Talk About Food*, American Medical Association, Chicago, 1970.
Student:
Showers, P., *What Happens to a Hamburger*, Crowell, New York, 1970.
Chapman, V.L., *Let's Go to the Supermarket*, Putnam, New York, 1972.
How Your Body Uses Food, National Dairy Council, Chicago.

Problem Area: *Environmental Health*   Grade: *5*

Title: *PROTECTING THE WORLD AROUND US*

Long Range Goal: *Conscientiously seeks to prevent pollution and protect the environment.*

Expected Outcomes
The student:
1. examines the nature and scope of the pollution problem.

276

2. identifies several categories of pollution.
3. explains the relationship between progress and pollution.
4. suggests various alternatives to protect the environment.
5. accepts a personal responsibility to protect the environment.
6. refrains from contributing to environmental pollution.

Content
*1. A. Ecology is the study of the relationship between living things and the environment.
   B. General terms to be defined include:
      (1) pollution.
      (2) food chain.
      (3) ecosystem.
2. A. Pollution exists in several forms.
   B. Categories of pollution include:
      (1) air.
      (2) water.
      (3) noise.
3. A. The industrial revolution and recent technological advances created much of the current pollution problem.
   B. Technological advancements have been partially responsible for problems such as:
      (1) increased industrial pollution.
      (2) prevalence of pesticides.
      (3) automobile emissions.
      (4) radiation hazards.
   C. Increased pollution has resulted in a rise in certain diseases.
   D. Population increases magnify the problems of pollution.
4. A. Legal action controls some forms of pollution.
   B. Voluntary efforts have reduced the pollution problem.
   C. Proper architectural design can lessen the effects of pollution.
5. A. Increased family size contributes to world population and pollution problems.
   B. Pollution can be partially controlled through ecology efforts in the home.
6. A. Waste materials should be disposed of properly.
   B. Open burning of trash is a source of pollution.
   C. Automobile emission equipment should be in proper working order.

* numbers refer to expected outcomes.

Methods
Study charts of food chains and food webs.
View a film or filmstrip on pollution.
Conduct laboratory tests for the presence of selected pollutants.
Invite a physician to discuss diseases related to pollution.
Design an ecology-oriented model community.
Complete an environmental improvement project at home or at school.
List sources of pollution at home or at school.

Plan a recycling project.
Visit a garage to observe automobile emission control equipment.
Inspect the local sanitary landfill.
Question a representative of the Environmental Protection Agency.
Debate merits of various pollution control measures.
Invite a sanitary engineer or sanitarian to discuss pollution.

Aids
Food chain charts
Pollution film or filmstrip
Laboratory pollution test kit
Environmental control equipment

Evaluation
Test
Observation
Project evaluation

References
Teacher:
Man and His Endangered World: ABC's of Human Ecology, Bete, Greenfield, Massachusetts, 1972.
Miles, B., *Save the Earth! An Ecology Handbook for Kids*, Knopf, New York, 1974.
Richmond, J.B. et al., *You and Your Health*, Orange Level Teacher's Edition, Scott Foresman, Glenview, Illinois, 1977.
Sorochan, W.D. and S.J. Bender, *Teaching Elementary Health Science*, Addison-Wesley, Reading, Massachusetts, 1975.
You Learn and Change, Teacher's Edition, Harcourt, Brace & Jovanovich, New York, 1977.
Student:
Kalina, S., *Three Drops of Water*, Lothrop Lee & Shepard, New York, 1974.
Pringle, L., *City and Suburb*, Macmillan, New York, 1975.
Shanks, A.Z., *About Garbage and Stuff*, Viking, New York, 1973.
Tannenbaum, B. and M. Stillman, *Clean Air*, McGraw-Hill, Hightstown, New Jersey, 1974.

Problem Area: *Emotional Health*   Grade: 7

Title: *UNDERSTANDING DEATH*

Long Range Goal: *Adjusts to the reality of death.*

Expected Outcomes
The student:
1. compares the American view of death with that of other societies.
2. understands the method in which Americans adjust to the concept of death.

3. examines the five psychological stages related to the acceptance of death.
4. realizes the extent of the suicide problem in the United States and the world.
5. acknowledges the importance of positive attitudes toward the death of oneself and others.
6. accepts the importance of death education.

Content
*1. A. The perception of death varies in countries throughout the world.
   B. Distinct views of death exist among:
      (1) Europeans.
      (2) Asians.
      (3) Africans.
2. A. Immortality is obtained through religion, work, or children.
   B. The American culture is oriented toward youth.
   C. Americans are shielded from the reality of death by:
      (1) unrealistic media representations.
      (2) assignment of the elderly to nursing homes.
   D. Children are not confronted with the reality of death.
   E. Funerals are conducted with the survivors in mind.
3. A. Distinct psychological reactions to the reality of death occur among individuals.
   B. Dr. Elisabeth Kübler-Ross identified the five psychological stages of:
      (1) denial.
      (2) anger.
      (3) bargaining.
      (4) depression.
      (5) acceptance.
4. A. Suicide is a problem for people of all ages.
   B. Young people may commit suicide.
   C. Reasons for suicide include stress, depression, and illness.
5. A. Individuals can adjust to the absence of a friend or relative who dies.
   B. The death of oneself represents the end of all reality and life.
6. A. All living organisms will die.
   B. Accepting death as a reality can help the individual fully appreciate the meaning of life.

* numbers refer to expected outcomes.

Methods
Prepare reports on the views of death held by other societies.
View a film or filmstrip on the death of a grandparent.
Conduct a survey on the cost of a funeral.
Invite qualified ministers to discuss the religious implications of death.
Survey the class to determine how many students have casually considered suicide and explore these feelings.
Discuss the feelings that result from the loss of a pet.
Discuss the feelings that result from the loss of a friend or relative.
List goals for the future for each student.

Aids
Film or filmstrip

Evaluation
Knowledge test
Report evaluation
Survey evaluation
Attitude scale

References
Teacher:
Grollman, E.A., *Explaining Death to Children*, Beacon, Boston, 1967.
Hart, E.J., and C.E. Kofoed, "A Resource Unit on Death Education: Part I," *Eta Sigma Gamman* 8:24–27, Spring, 1976.
Hart, E.J. and C.E. Kofoed, "A Resource Unit on Death Education: Part II," *Eta Sigma Gamman* 8:10–15, Autumn, 1976.
Hendin, D., *Death as a Fact of Life*, Warner, New York, 1974.
Jackson, E.N., *Telling a Child About Death*, Hawthorne, New York, 1965.
Kübler-Ross, E., *On Death and Dying*, Macmillan, New York, 1969.
Schwartz, S., "Death Education: Suggested Readings and Audiovisuals," *Journal of School Health* 47:607–609, December, 1977.
Vogel, L.J., *Helping a Child Understand Death*, Fortress, Philadelphia, 1975.
Student:
Irwin, T.K., "Marcia's Walk Through the Valley of the Shadow," *Family Weekly*, May 20, 1973.
Kübler-Ross, E., *Questions and Answers on Death and Dying*, Macmillan, New York, 1974.
"When You Lose a Loved One," Public Affairs Commission, New York.

Problem Area: *Mood Modifying Substances*   Grade: *9*

Title: *THINKING ABOUT DRINKING?*

Long Range Goal: *Understands the dangers of drug abuse and does not abuse drugs.*

Expected Outcomes
The student:
1. traces the history of the use of alcohol.
2. evaluates reasons for the consumption of alcohol.
3. understands the effects of alcohol on the body.
4. examines the problem of alcoholism.
5. realizes the reasons for laws regulating the consumption of alcohol.
6. accepts the need for consuming alcohol in moderation.

Content
*1. A.   Alcohol was historically consumed in religious ceremonies and social customs.
   B.   Efforts to control alcohol consumption in the United States included:
      (1) Prohibition.
      (2) Women's Christian Temperance Union.
      (3) local and state legislation.
2. A.   Adult consumption of alcohol is influenced by:
      (1) economic level.
      (2) social factors.
      (3) health status.
   B.   Alcohol consumption among young people is influenced by peer pressure and family factors.
   C.   Advertising of alcohol promotes its consumption.
3. A.   Alcohol consumption may result in organic damage to include:
      (1) impaired respiration.
      (2) digestive disturbances.
      (3) nervous disorders.
      (4) urinary problems.
      (5) circulatory damage.
   B.   Alcohol may impair:
      (1) vision.
      (2) speech.
      (3) coordination.
      (4) judgment.
      (5) memory.
      (6) social interaction.
   C.   Chronic disorders related to alcohol consumption develop over extended periods of time.
4. A.   The problem of alcoholism exists throughout the world.
   B.   The alcoholic causes specific problems within the community.
   C.   Home and family life is seriously affected by the alcoholic.
   D.   Stress and pressure are significant factors in the development of alcoholism.
   E.   Programs such as Alcoholics Anonymous provide the most effective means of treatment.
   F.   Preventing alcoholism is much easier than treating it.
5. A.   Specific regulations controlling the sale and consumption of alcohol exist at the:
      (1) local level.
      (2) state level.
      (3) federal level.
   B.   Specific penalties for violation of the regulations exist at each level.
6. A.   Several methods may be utilized to control the amount of alcohol consumed.
   B.   Consumption of alcohol involves certain personal responsibility to oneself and others.

* numbers refer to expected outcomes.

Methods
Prepare a report on the historical uses of alcohol.
Invite a WCTU representative to speak to the class.
Review various advertisements for alcoholic beverages.
Simulate physical impairments resulting from alcohol consumption.
View a film or filmstrip on the reasons for consuming alcohol.
Conduct a panel discussion on the pro and con aspects of alcohol consumption.
Visit an open meeting of Alcoholics Anonymous.
Invite a reformed alcoholic to speak to the class.

Aids
Sources of advertisements
Film or filmstrip
AV equipment
Simulation props

Evaluation
Knowledge test
Attitude scale
Observation
Report evaluation
Practice inventory

References
Teacher:
Block, M.A., *Alcohol and Alcoholism,* Wadsworth, Belmont, California, 1970.
Carroll, C.R., *Alcohol: Use, Nonuse, and Abuse,* Brown, Dubuque, Iowa, 1975.
Hafen, B.Q., *Alcohol: The Crutch That Cripples,* West, Saint Paul, 1977.
Jones, K.L., and others, *Drugs: Substance Abuse,* Canfield, San Francisco, 1975.
Student:
Hall, L.C., *Facts About Alcohol and Alcoholism,* National Institute on Alcohol Abuse and Alcoholism, Rockville, Maryland, 1975.
McCarthy, R.G., *Facts About Alcohol,* (revised by J.J. Pasciutti), Science Research Associates, Chicago, 1967.
Miles, S.A., *Learning About Alcohol,* American Alliance for Health, Physical Education, and Recreation, Washington, 1974.
Needle, R.H. and A.E. Hill, *Basic Concepts of Alcohol,* Laidlaw, River Forest, Illinois, 1972.
Saltman, J., *The New Alcoholics: Teenagers,* No. 499, Public Affairs Pamphlets, New York, 1973.
The Drinking Game and How to Beat It, No. 456, Children's Bureau, Washington, 1968.

Problem Area: *Marriage and Family Living*　　　　　　　　　　　　　　　　Grade: *11*

Title: *THINKING ABOUT GETTING MARRIED?*

Long Range Goal: *Accepts the responsibility of behaving as a good family member.*

Expected Outcomes

The student:

1. reviews the history of marriage in the United States.
2. lists advantages and disadvantages to remaining unmarried.
3. explores social and moral aspects of the marriage relationship.
4. realizes that marriage requires personal maturity.
5. appreciates the unique roles played by various family members.
6. displays tolerance toward the problems of other family members.

Content

*1. A. Current marital practices are influenced by history.
   B. Historically, marriage in the United States:
     (1) established the family unit.
     (2) provided financial security.
     (3) conformed to existing social patterns.
     (4) promoted reproduction.
     (5) supported prevalent religious beliefs.

2. A. Remaining unmarried has advantages and disadvantages.
   B. Specific advantages and disadvantages include:
     (1) increased professional mobility.
     (2) extended sexual relations.
     (3) lower comparable income.
     (4) living on a single income.
     (5) housing restrictions.
     (6) job preference for married individuals.

3. A. Social and moral responsibilities include:
     (1) requirements of society.
     (2) personal responsibility to and for a mate.
     (3) concern for children.
   B. Mutual satisfaction of needs is a prime responsibility in marriage.

4. A. Maturity is an important aspect of a successful marriage.
   B. Personal maturity includes:
     (1) emotional stability.
     (2) social stability.
     (3) self-discipline.
     (4) unselfishness.
     (5) money management skills.
     (6) healthy sexual adjustment.

5. A. Society prescribes traditional family roles for:
     (1) father.
     (2) mother.
     (3) children.
     (4) siblings.
     (5) other relatives.

* numbers refer to expected outcomes.

B. Role variations occur based upon the individual needs and circumstances of each family.
C. Conflict may occur when role definitions blur or overlap.
6. A. Each family member experiences unique problems due to role requirements.
B. Tolerance and understanding reduce family role conflicts.

Methods
Report on early courtship and marriage practices in the United States.
Conduct a home survey to list advantages to marriage.
Invite a family counselor to discuss social and moral aspects of marriage.
Plan a sample budget for a recently married couple.
List the functions of various family members.
Role-play the functions of various family members.
Employ problem solving to resolve a number of hypothetical conflicts involving family members.
Suggest a number of possibilities for enjoyable family outings.

Aids
Home survey form
Budget planning sheet
Role-playing props

Evaluation
Test
Report evaluation
Project evaluation
Observation

References
Teacher:
Burt, J.J. and L.B. Meeks, *Toward A Health Sexuality*, Saunders, Philadelphia, 1973.
Growth Patterns and Sex Education, American School Health Association, Kent, Ohio, 1967.
Jones, K.L. et al., *Sex*, Second Edition, Harper and Row, New York, 1973.
McCary, J.L., *Freedom and Growth in Marriage*, Hamilton, Santa Barbara, California, 1975.
Student:
11 Million Teenagers, Alan Guttmacher Institute, New York, 1976.
Johnson, E.W., *Sex: Telling it Straight*, Bantam, Philadelphia, 1971.
Wood, A., *The Seventeen Book of Answers to What Your Parents Don't Talk About*, McKay, New York, 1972.

Problem Area: *Emotional Health*   Grade: *College*

Title: *COPING WITH EMOTIONAL STRESS*

Long Range Goal: *Analyzes the nature and source of stress and copes with it successfully.*

Expected Outcomes
The student:
1. understands the physiological effects of stress.
2. identifies potential sources of stress affecting the college student.
3. examines alternatives in coping with stressful situations.
4. realizes the importance of self-confidence in coping with stress.
5. appreciates the necessity of accepting self and others.
6. attempts to deal more effectively with stress.

Content
*1. A. Physiological changes result from continued stress.
   B. Stress causes physiological changes in the:
     (1) digestive system.
     (2) circulatory system.
     (3) nervous system.
2. A. A variety of circumstances may generate stress.
   B. Specific sources of stress include:
     (1) scholastic pressure.
     (2) fatigue.
     (3) aftermath of physical illness.
     (4) negative romantic experiences.
     (5) conflicting values.
3. A. Alternatives to stress include:
     (1) increased physical activity.
     (2) formal and informal health counseling.
     (3) improved personal health practices.
     (4) value clarification.
     (5) meaningful spiritual life.
   B. Much stress is self-induced.
   C. Harmful health practices such as smoking and heavy alcohol consumption aggravate stressful situations.
4. A. Individuals must personally analyze their own life-styles to identify the causes of stress.
   B. Each alternative to stress has advantages and disadvantages depending on the individual.
   C. Self-concept influences the manner in which the individual views life.
5. A. Each individual possesses limitations that must be accepted.
   B. Acceptance of personal limitations increases tolerance of the limitations of others.
   C. A negative attitude toward others is an individual ego-protection mechanism.
6. A. A personal decision to overcome specific causes of stress is the first step in effectively coping with stress.
   B. Avoiding potentially stressful situations when possible is helpful.

* numbers refer to expected outcomes.

Methods
Demonstrate the effect of an unexpected loud noise on heart rate and blood pressure.
Brainstorm a collection of potentially stressful situations affecting the college student.
Role-play various alternatives to a number of hypothetical situations involving stress.
Utilize a number of value clarification exercises.
Determine the effect of cigarette smoking on heart rate and blood pressure.
Complete a personality and self-concept inventory.
Invite a psychologist or counselor to speak to the class.

Aids
Noise device
Role playing props
Cigarettes
Blood pressure gauge
Personality inventory

Evaluation
Knowledge test
Observation
Behavior inventory
Attitude scale

References
Teacher:
Bower, E.M., *Teachers Talk About Their Feelings*, National Institute of Mental Health, Rockville, Maryland, 1973.
Jones, K.L. et al., *Emotional Health*, Second Edition, Canfield Press, San Francisco, 1975.
Mental Health at School, National Institute of Mental Health, Rockville, Maryland, 1973.
Samuels, H., *Mental Health,* Brown, Dubuque, Iowa, 1975.
Student:
A Consumer's Guide to Mental Health Services, National Institute of Mental Health, Rockville, Maryland, 1975.
How to Deal with Mental Problems, National Association for Mental Health, New York.
Mental Illness and Its Treatment, National Institute of Mental Health, Rockville, Maryland, 1972.
Some Things You Should Know About Mental and Emotional Illness, National Association for Mental Health, Arlington, Virginia.

Problem Area: *Family Living*   Grade: *Early Adult*

Title: *SO, I'M A PARENT!*

Long Range Goal: *Understands and accepts the responsibilities of being a parent.*

286

Expected Outcomes

The Student:

1. identifies the cost involved in having a baby.
2. understands that a parent must provide the child with certain daily needs.
3. practices proper daily care requirements of a baby.
4. realizes that certain social adjustments are necessary after having a baby.
5. accepts that a new baby may create emotional stress between new parents.
6. appreciates that successful parenthood is influenced by a proper attitude.

Contents

1. A. Actual delivery expenses include:
      (1) physician fees.
      (2) hospital charges.
      (3) medication costs.
   B. Related expenses include:
      (1) baby clothes, furniture, and accessories.
      (2) maternity wardrobe.
      (3) special insurance policies.
2. A. The baby must be fed at regular intervals.
   B. Diapers must be changed as necessary.
   C. Baby clothes and diapers must be washed and ironed.
   D. Safety precautions must be taken to protect the baby.
   E. Parents should play with and hold the baby.
3. A. Baby food must be prepared in a sanitary manner.
   B. Appropriate types of food must be selected for a new baby.
   C. The baby must be burped after eating.
   D. The baby must be periodically bathed in a safe and proper fashion.
   E. Diapers must be removed and replaced properly.
4. A. A baby affects the social life of the parents.
   B. Social adjustments resulting from having a baby include:
      (1) reduced flexibility and personal freedom.
      (2) restricted social activities.
      (3) loss of commonality with childless friends.
5. A. A baby may cause emotional stress between parents.
   B. Emotional stress between new parents may result from:
      (1) lack of time alone for communication.
      (2) jealousy from the necessity to share attention and affection.
      (3) having to give primary attention to the needs of the baby.
      (4) increased financial pressure.
      (5) fatigue.
6. A. Couples should honestly share their feelings about prospective parenthood.
   B. Positive attitudes toward parenthood should be identified, studied, and discussed.
   C. Positive initial attitudes toward parenthood increase the probability of success.

D. Improper attitudes toward parenthood may lead to poor adjustment to the baby, conflicts with the spouse, mistreatment of the baby, and related problems.

Methods
Survey physicians, hospitals, and new parents to determine the direct and indirect costs of having a baby.
Conduct a field trip to a child day care center.
Demonstrate the proper method of changing a diaper.
Demonstrate the proper method of feeding a baby.
Demonstrate the proper method of bathing a baby.
Question parents concerning the changes parenthood made in their lives.
Invite two new parents to discuss the social and emotional changes resulting from parenthood.
Invite a pediatrician to discuss child care procedures.
Request information on child abuse from Parents Anonymous.
Invite an insurance representative to discuss insurance plans.

Aids
Doll (or baby)
Diapers (cloth and disposable)
Safety pins
Baby powder
Tissues
Baby bath
Towels
Baby bottle
Milk or formula
Baby food
Utensils
Bib

Evaluation
Knowledge test
Observation
Project evaluation
Attitude scale

References (Teacher/Student)
DeFrancis, V., *The Fundamentals of Child Protection*, American Humane Association, Denver, 1955.
Dreikurs, R., *Children: The Challenge*, Hawthorne, New York, 1964.
Gilberg, A., "The Stress of Parenting," *Child Psychiatry and Human Development*, 6:59–67, Winter, 1975.
Gordon, T., *Parent Effectiveness Training*, Wyden, New York, 1970.
Klemer, R.H., *Marriage and Family Relationships*, Harper and Row, New York, 1970.

McCary, J.L., *Freedom and Growth in Marriage*, Hamilton, Santa Barbara, California, 1975.

Salk, L., *What Every Child Would Like His Parents to Know*, McKay, New York, 1972.

Skolnick, A.S. and J.H. Skolnick, *Family in Transition*, Little Brown, Boston, 1971.

Problem Area: *Health in the Middle Years*   Grade: *Middle Adult*

Title: *RECOGNIZING EARLY SIGNS OF ILLNESS*

Long Range Goal: *Understands the early signs of illness and responds to them intelligently.*

Expected Outcomes

The student:

1. realizes that prevention of health problems is preferable to treatment of the problems.
2. understands what signs and symptoms of illness warrant the consultation of a physician.
3. learns the signs and symptoms of cancer.
4. examines physical factors that may lead to heart disease.
5. knows the signs and symptoms of diabetes.
6. visits the family physician when signs or symptoms indicate a deviation from normal health.

Content

1. A. Prevention of certain health problems may be accomplished through measures such as:
    (1) proper diet.
    (2) adequate rest.
    (3) regular exercise.
    (4) moderate use of alcohol.
    (5) refraining from smoking.
    (6) control of stress factors.
   B. Failure to practice prevention may result in a number of serious and costly health problems.

2. A. A physician should be consulted when:
    (1) the person is in intense pain.
    (2) symptoms exist for an extended period.
    (3) symptoms periodically recur.
    (4) a serious accident or emergency situation occurs.
    (5) the person is worried about the condition.
   B. Some specific situations requiring the consultation of a physician include:
    (1) serious bleeding.
    (2) lack of breathing.
    (3) shock.
    (4) poisoning.

(5) serious infection.

(6) bone fractures.

(7) chest pain.

(8) persistent diarrhea and vomiting.

(9) mental disorientation.

(10) drug reactions.

(11) continuous high fever.

3. A. Early detection of cancer is important for effective treatment.

   B. The American Cancer Society's seven warning signals of cancer are:

   (1) a sore that fails to heal.

   (2) changes in bowel or bladder habits.

   (3) unusual bleeding or discharge.

   (4) thickening or lump in the breast or elsewhere.

   (5) noticeable change in a wart or mole.

   (6) indigestion or difficulty swallowing.

   (7) persistent cough or hoarseness.

4. A. Factors contributing to heart disease include:

   (1) improper nutrition and obesity.

   (2) inadequate exercise.

   (3) smoking.

   (4) uncontrolled stress.

   (5) high blood pressure.

   B. Symptoms of heart disease may include:

   (1) severe chest pain.

   (2) pain extending into the neck or arm.

   (3) nausea and vomiting.

   (4) sweating.

   (5) shortness of breath.

   (6) loss of consciousness.

5. A. Factors contributing to diabetes include:

   (1) family history of diabetes.

   (2) age over forty.

   (3) obesity.

   B. Treatment of diabetes involves:

   (1) use of medication.

   (2) modification of diet.

   (3) regular exercise.

6. A. Routine medical examinations should include evaluation of:

   (1) personal and family health histories.

   (2) routine and special laboratory tests.

   (3) results of the physical examination by the physician.

   B. Routine medical examinations lessen the worry over individual health and reduce the risk of death and disease.

Methods

Invite a physician to discuss the question of when to consult a physician.

Distribute literature from the American Cancer Society.
Discuss the cause and prevention of cancer with a representative of the American Cancer Society.
View a film or filmstrip concerning heart disease.
Practice measuring blood pressure and pulse rate.
Obtain literature from the American Heart Association.
Question a diabetic individual concerning procedures to control the disease.
Examine literature related to diabetes.
Study forms, laboratory reports, and other materials related to a medical examination.
Invite a physician to discuss medical examinations.

Aids
Cancer literature
Heart literature
Diabetes literature
Film or filmstrip
Projection equipment
Sample medical examination report
Blood pressure gauge

Evaluation
Knowledge test
Attitude scale
Observation
Practice inventory

References (Teacher/Student)
Benenson, A.S., *Control of Communicable Diseases in Man*, 12th Ed., American Public Health Association, New York, 1975.
Friedman, M. and R.H. Rosenman, *Type A Behavior and Your Heart*, Knopf, New York, 1974.
Levin, L.S. et al., *Self Care: Lay Initiatives in Health*, Prodist, New York, 1976.
Schifferes, J.J., *The Family Medical Encyclopedia*, Pocket, New York, 1959.
Schnert, K.W. with H. Eisenberg, *How to be Your Own Doctor (Sometimes)*, Grossett and Dunlap, New York, 1976.
Sheehy, G., *Passages: Predictable Crises of Adult Life*, Dutton, New York, 1977.
When to Call or See Your Physician and other publications, American Medical Association, Chicago.
"When to Call the Doctor" in *Today's Health Guide*, W.W. Bauer, editor, American Medical Association, Chicago, 1965.
Vickery, D.M. and J.F. Fries, *Take Care of Yourself: A Consumer's Guide to Medical Care*, Addison-Wesley, Reading, Massachusetts, 1976.

Problem Area: *Health of the Older Adult*   Grade: *Older Adult*

Title: *NUTRITION IN RETIREMENT*

Long Range Goal: *Understands and implements measures to conserve health.*

Expected Outcomes
The student:
1. understands the special dietary requirements of older persons.
2. identifies various factors that influence life span.
3. analyzes procedures related to effective food shopping practices.
4. realizes that a number of factors affect proper nutritional practices.
5. plans simple and nutritious meals.

Content
1. A. Extended life expectancies in countries other than the United States relate to:
     (1) lack of pollution.
     (2) rural life-style.
     (3) attitude toward long life.
     (4) dietary practices.
     (5) low levels of stress.
   B. The diet of individuals in such countries generally consist of fewer calories and lower levels of animal fat than the American diet.
2. A. Specific practices promoting extended life span include:
     (1) reduction in caloric intake.
     (2) reduction in salt intake.
     (3) moderate consumption of alcohol.
     (4) refraining from smoking.
     (5) control of weight.
     (6) regular exercise.
     (7) reduction of stress.
   B. Cardiovascular diseases such as arteriosclerosis and atherosclerosis are related to factors of diet and exercise.
3. A. A proper diet for an older person should include:
     (1) high levels of protein.
     (2) bread and grain products.
     (3) fresh fruits and vegetables.
     (4) milk and dairy products.
     (5) adequate amounts of fluids.
     (6) adequate amounts of fiber.
     (7) low fat intake.
     (8) low salt intake.
     (9) moderate caloric intake.
   B. Nutrient supplements may be prescribed for an older person by the attending physician.
4. A. Certain advertising approaches do not provide older consumers with accurate, objective information.
   B. Purchasing foods in appropriate quantities lessens problems of preparation and storage.

C. Labeling of food products provides nutritional information concerning:
   (1) vitamins.
   (2) minerals.
   (3) fat.
   (4) carbohydrates.
   (5) protein.
   (6) sodium.
   (7) additives.
5. A. Living conditions may affect the ability of older persons to regularly prepare nutritious meals.
   B. General health problems may prevent older persons from maintaining an adequate diet.
   C. Various health, welfare, and charitable agencies and organizations provide meals for older persons needing assistance.
   D. Kitchen safety practices should be carefully maintained.
   E. Foods must be properly stored.
6. A. Selecting foods from the four food groups is essential for a balanced diet.
   B. Adequate amounts of fiber and fluids must be consumed.
   C. Highly processed convenience foods are often of questionable nutritional value.

Methods
Review case studies of individuals experiencing a long life span.
Examine the diets of several countries with high levels of health and long life expectancies.
Invite a nutritionist to discuss the elements of a balanced diet for older persons.
Analyze various advertisements for health and food products.
Collect a sample of various sizes of food containers and packages.
Study nutrition labels on several food products.
Identify local agencies and organizations giving assistance to older people.
Demonstrate kitchen safety practices.
Plan and serve a series of simple, nutritious meals and snacks.
Discuss exercise and general health practices of older persons with a gerontologist.

Aids
Reference materials on life span
Advertisements
Food containers and packages
Nutrition labels
Kitchen utensils
Cookbooks

Evaluation
Observation
Discussion
Project evaluation

Checklist
Practice inventory

References (Teacher/Student)
Food Facts Talk Back and other publications, American Dietetic Association, Chicago.
Goodhart, R.S. and M.E. Shils, *Modern Nutrition in Health and Disease*, Lea & Febiger, Philadelphia, 1973.
Mayer, J., *Overweight, Causes, Cost, and Control*, Prentice-Hall, Englewood Cliffs, New Jersey, 1968.
Nutrition Books, evaluative review, Chicago Nutrition Association, Chicago.
Whanger, A.D., "Vitamins and Vigor at 65 Plus," *Postgraduate Medicine*, February, 1973, p. 167.
White, P.L., *Let's Talk About Food*, American Medical Association, Chicago, 1970.
Williams, R.J., *Nutrition in a Nutshell*, Doubleday, Garden City, New York, 1976.
Your Age and Your Diet and other publications, American Medical Association, Chicago.

Index